WRINKLES

How to Prevent Them,
How to Erase Them

by Lida Livingston
and Constance Schrader

Prentice-Hall, Inc., Englewood Cliffs, New Jersey

To Julie, who thought of it all.
To Lida, a loving friend.

Photographs by Payneshots:
Exercise pictures of Faith Catlin
Face background picture of Deinse Hillhouse

Wrinkles: How to Prevent Them, How to Erase Them
by Lida Livingston and Constance Schrader
Copyright © 1978 by Lida Livingston and Constance Schrader

Printed in the United States of America
Prentice-Hall International, Inc., London/Prentice-Hall of Australia, Pty. Ltd., Sydney/ Prentice-Hall of Canada, Ltd., Toronto/Prentice-Hall of India Private Ltd., New Delhi/ Prentice-Hall of Japan, Inc., Tokyo/Prentice-Hall of Southeast Asia Pte. Ltd., Singapore/ Whitehall Books Limited, Wellington, New Zealand
10 9 8 7 6 5 4 3 2 1

Library of Congress Cataloging in Publication Data

Livingston, Lida, 1912-1977.
  Wrinkles: how to prevent them, how to erase them.

  Bibliography: p.
    1. Skin—Care and hygiene.   2.   Skin—Wrinkles.
I.   Schrader, Constance, joint author.
II.   Title
RL87.L58   646.7'26   78-3858
ISBN 0-13-970186-9

Acknowledgements

At first we tried to keep a list of all the people who were of help to us in gathering the information, typing, consulting with us, and even testing the methods described. The list nears a hundred people. And they were all of great help.

Thanks to everyone! To the doctors and dentists who freely gave of their time and advice and provided specific knowledge, to the nimble fingers of Jean Brown, our typist, who read copy that was unreadable, to our editors and art directors, and to the photographers and models who labored to capture the problems and the beauty of skin.

To our relatives and friends who were helpful and supportive.

> ''*Beauty is Nature's coin, must not be hoarded,*
> *But must be current, and the good thereof*
> *Consist in mutual and partaken bliss . . .*''

Milton, *Comus*

Contents

Preface

Wrinkles afflict most of the female population over 25. They are the number one beauty anxiety. This book is dedicated to helping those of you who have wrinkles turn back the clock, and to helping stave off wrinkles for those of you so young, you do not have a single one. That usually means you're on the sunny side of 21. Twenty-one is not too young to initiate your anti-wrinkle campaign. It's even better to start younger. But, while prevention is always preferable to cure, this book will help you if you're 40, 60, 80 or even more. It's never too late to be more beautiful.

Beauty depends on six things only:

1. Cleanliness—ridding the skin of soil and dead cells.
2. What you put into your body.
3. What you put on your body—on your skin and your hair.
4. If and how you exercise your body, including your face.
5. If and how you massage your body, including your face.
6. What you think.

Number six is the key.

Everything you think shows on your face. What you think about yourself shows in the shape of your body, the condition of your skin and hair, and the clothes you wear.

Abraham Lincoln was once chided for refusing a man a job.

"Didn't like his face," said Lincoln.

"You can't refuse a man a job because you don't like his face!" came the protest.

"I can," Lincoln retorted. "He's over 40. After 40, a man's *responsible* for his face!"

This story was told to the great film and stage director, Rouben Mamoulian, who guided Greta Garbo, Tyrone Power, and other luminaries in such unforgettable films as *Ninotchka* and *Blood and Sand*, and directed a number of stage classics, including the original *Porgy and Bess*.

"Lincoln was right," Mamoulian said, "but he had the age wrong. A person is responsible for his face from 20 on."

A happy thought is that, regardless of your age and previous facial irresponsibility, from today on you can start having your face say positive things about you.

Author's Note

The methods, products, and techniques described in this book have been thoroughly tested by the authors and other beauty experts. Every person is unique, however, and common sense and ordinary caution should be used in applying these methods, products, and techniques to find out if they work for each individual.

Part One

FIRST STEPS

One

WRINKLES AND THEIR CAUSES

"The flowers anew, returning seasons bring!
But beauty faded has no second spring."

Ambrose Philips

When Ambrose Philips wrote that back in the early eighteenth century, he had no knowledge of the miracles that can be wrought by the body's cells and muscles and circulation, particularly when tethered to the will of a woman determined upon her right to be beautiful.

The clock can be turned back. Changes in face and body and figure can be achieved—and without recourse to surgery.

The surgeon's knife has reversed time for a period of five to ten years for countless thousands, but the reversal is only temporary and the turn-back must be harnessed to a personal action program to keep the years—the wrinkles, sags, and pouches—at bay. And that's what this book is all about: how to prevent wrinkles—which is easiest—and how to get rid of wrinkles—which is harder, but possible.

Most people consider wrinkles inevitable, along with death and taxes. But, in truth, the majority of wrinkles that occur are due not to inevitability but to three basic causes: ignorance, carelessness, and neglect.

Having taken for granted that wrinkles are inescapable, few women, and far fewer men, have ever investigated the causes of wrinkles, or their prevention.

3

The causes are many, including:

Faulty diet—a diet that is inadequate or lacking in the
   essential nutrients and in the particular nutrients that
   keep the skin looking fresh and glowing.
The elements—wind, and, most wickedly when it's not
   treated with respect, the sun.

A variety of facial mannerisms and other bad habits, including:

Wrinkling the forehead by way of verbal emphasis, or,
   similarly, lifting the eyebrows, which also puts wrinkles
   into the forehead.
Quirking one eyebrow to express skepticism or amused
   tolerance.
Sitting with chin in hand, thereby pushing wrinkles into
   one cheek.
Pulling the lips down in a grimace.
Scowling, pursing the lips, and frowning.
Talking out of one side of the mouth.

Also, of course, heredity is a factor: fair-skinned, red-haired, or fair-haired people wrinkle the most readily. Other causes include:

Tension, anger, and anxiety—stress of any kind.
Cigarette smoking, the villain behind many cases of
   crow's feet.
A malfunctioning liver.
Poor elimination.
A number of diseases, including, often, diabetes, now the
   nation's number three killer.
Inactivity of the inner muscles, leading to atrophy, hollows,
   and sagging.
The pull of gravity without counteraction.
Inadequate nourishment for the outer skin.
Inadequate water on the skin and in diet.
Certain ''creams'' and ''oils,'' soaps and shampoos that
   actually leach out nature's moisture and oil instead of
   contributing to it.

Facial masks that pull and stretch delicate skin tissue.
Tight shoes!
Thick pillows.

There are unknown causes too. Many dermatologists and other doctors consider wrinkles as something of a mystery. Some nutritionally minded doctors place the blame on diet, claiming that not only is a good diet required to counteract wrinkles, but perhaps vitamin and mineral supplementation as well. Actually, diet is vitally important, but exercise and ''smoothings'' are more so. Our smoothing program will:

1. Show results in a short period of time.
2. Not harm you in any way.
3. Not require the purchase of special creams or expensive equipment.
4. Be suitable to do at home, traveling, or anyplace.

These wrinkle-erasing techniques cannot stop time, but they can—without drugs, without caustic peelers, and without pain—allow you to have healthy, glowing, sleek, and vital skin throughout your life, at any age. The techniques will make the skin cells grow, cause the skin to exfoliate more rapidly, and make the skin appear and actually be more youthful.

The program works because it attacks wrinkles from *within* and *without*, in the following manner:

FROM THE INSIDE

1. Good nutrition.
2. Good elimination.

FROM THE OUTSIDE, WHERE THE WRINKLES ARE

1. Firming exercises that strengthen muscles.
2. Exercises that bring cleansing and nourishing blood to the surface.
3. Contouring exercises to eliminate defects, from hollow cheeks to double chins.

4. Plumping exercises that give the look of health.
5. Smoothing techniques that:
   Reinforce the benefits of exercise.
   Stimulate circulation.
   Force cream into the skin.
   Actually erase wrinkles.

You can have a more beautiful skin starting with the ten-day crash plan that will set you on your way to being wrinkle free. It's fun and easy. The supermarket is your beauty pantry. No chemicals, special creams, or costly devices are required. In your own home, with this book, you can start immediately. Make your kitchen, your bathroom, or your bedroom your beauty salon.

Special features of the book include:

1. A personalized approach. You make the choices of the foods you eat, the products you use, the wrinkles you erase.
2. Facial/body ''maps'' so that you can be your own beauty analyst.
3. Questionnaires so that you can identify every wrinkle and analyze your skin care/beauty treatment routines, and improve them as you choose.
4. Information about alternative approaches.
5. Formulas for skin care products you can make yourself as well as a resource list of commercially available products.
6. A multi-faceted program of skin cleansing, nourishment, massage, and ''smoothings''; exercises for your face and body; nutrition with emphasis on ''beauty foods''— a *total* program so you can say goodbye to wrinkles.

Two

WHEN AND WHERE WRINKLES APPEAR

The onset of wrinkles may be delayed, but eventually time will tell—unless you take preventive action. Everyone's skin passes through specific conditions. No one can tell exactly when which wrinkles will appear, but Dr. Herbert J. Spoor, a New York dermatologist, has summarized the depressing picture as follows:

> At 20 years: The facial skin is free of wrinkles, the cheeks are rounded, so that the mouth and nose appear small.
>
> At 25 years: Forehead and often lower lids show the first signs. "Laugh lines" become apparent.
>
> At 30 years: Lateral lines appear at the outer edges of the eyes; crow's-feet can appear.
>
> At 35 years: Folds appear in front of the ears. Hair often begins to turn gray.
>
> At 40 years: Bags and wrinkles appear at the side of the mouth and under the eyes.
>
> At 45 years: Double chin appears; the lips become thinner and the eyebrows appear bushy.
>
> At 50 years: Wrinkles appear on bridge of nose, earlobes, and chin. Skin appears to be dry.
>
> At 55 years: Folds appear on the neck and at the nape of the neck.
>
> At 60 years: Cheeks have begun to sag. Teeth appear longer because gums have begun to recede.

At 65 years: There is hair growth in ear canals, in nostrils, and on neck.

At 70 years: Wrinkles crease over each other to form nets. The scalp hair is thin if not absent.

WHERE ARE YOUR WRINKLES?

Where wrinkles and hollows form earliest depends very much on the shape of your face.

If you have a narrow jaw and face, you are prone to vertical nose-to-chin lines and center cheek hollows.

If you have a broad jaw and face, your cheeks may look quite smooth from the front, but in profile you may notice hollows behind the cheeks as the face narrows back toward the ears.

The broad-jawed person is more prone to double chin development.

Each of these problems can be prevented, or corrected to a major extent, by friction (exercise) and ''smoothings,'' even to redevelopment of the round jaw of youth. Alternating contraction/relaxation exercise and using deep massage stimulate the muscles and the circulation of blood through the vessels and capillaries that nourish muscle and skin tissue. Like a piece of leather, the skin smooths as it is polished with oil or cream, along with deep massage.

Exercise strengthens and enlarges muscles of the face, neck, and throat just as it does elsewhere on the body. The problem is that no one ever taught most of us the value of facial exercise and so we simply ignored these muscles so vital to the impression we create.

Ninon de Lenclos, the astonishing seventeenth-century Frenchwoman who captivated the brilliant minds of France throughout her life, apparently needed no teacher and developed face and throat exercises for herself that made her a celebrated beauty until she died in 1706, at the age of 90 years and six months. When she was 85, Louis XIV called her ''the marvel'' of his reign. A pamphlet giving some of her exercises was published in 1710 by Jeanne Sauval, who for more than half a century was Mlle. de Lenclos's personal and faithful attendant. The message of the book was: Mlle. de Lenclos did it. You can do it too. In another old book, she was described as follows:

> ''Ninon's form was as symmetrical, elegant and yielding as a willow; her complexion of a dazzling white, with sparkling eyes as black as midnight; her teeth like pearls, her mouth mobile, her smile captivating and resistless. Adorable as she was in youth so she continued to be until her death. An incredible fact, but so well attested by the greatest and most reliable writers who testify to the truth of it that there is no reason to doubt.
> ''Ninon attributed it not to any miracle or natural traits, but to her philosophy (that is, her methods of physical and facial preservation), and declared that any one might exhibit the same peculiarities by following the same precepts.''

She also generously taught her techniques to friends, as the biography also noted:

> ''We have it on the most undoubted testimony of contemporaneous writers who were intimate with him that one of her dearest friends and followers, Saint Evremond, at the age of 89 years, inspired one of the famous beauties of the English court with an ardent attachment.''

In addition to the facial exercises included in this book, you can make up your own, as Ninon de Lenclos did. You cannot contract and relax facial muscles without increasing circulation. This releases fresh building material to rebuild worn-out tissues and combats wrinkles.

Three

🌿YOUR BEAUTY QUESTIONNAIRES🌿

Take a piece of loose-leaf paper, and as you read the questionnaires that follow, write down the appropriate answers. Thus you will create a ''Beauty Profile'' worksheet for yourself. You'll note there is no suggestion that you put down your age, as there always is in medical questionnaries. Your skin has its own age.

Keep your worksheet, and others based on questionnaires elsewhere in the book, in a loose-leaf folder, which will be a record for yourself of the problems or annoyances that you want to get rid of. After you fill out each questionnaire, we suggest you set a specific goal, or goals, designed to stimulate you into undertaking steps to improve your health and prevent or reduce wrinkles. You may want to create a general goal, such as: ''To attack these problems, and overcome them,'' or one or more specific goals, perhaps related to a single wrinkle or beauty fault.

Keep your worksheet private but *keep* it—for the sense of satisfaction you'll feel when you have overcome your problems. Date each worksheet. When conditions improve, it's easy to forget the things that once worried you.

Your Skin Questionnaire

Closely examine your skin. Is it:	*Never*	*Usually*	*Always*
Dewy, glowing?	✓		
Smooth, unlined, with a soft pliable covering?	✓		

11

	n	u	a
Rough-dry?		✓	
Scaly, flaky?		✓	
Bumpy, with small deposits under the skin?	✓		
Fine textured and unlined?	✓		
Wrinkled?		✓	
Blotchy?		✓	
Marred with brown spots?		✓	
Marred with moles?		✓	
Thin, shiny?			
Greasy?		✓	
Large pored?		✓	
Pimpled?		✓	

Are sections of your face and neck dry, or oily? If so, note:

	Dry	Oily	Normal
Forehead		✓	
Eyes			✓
Nose		✓	
Mouth			✓
Cheeks			✓
Temples		✓	
Chin			✓
Throat			✓
Shoulders		✓	
Back of neck		✓	

	Yes	No
Does your skin bruise easily?		✓
Does your skin heal quickly after minor cuts or wounds?		✓
Does your skin scar easily?	✓	
Do marks and discolorations from bruises last longer than a few weeks?		✓
Can you see the pores in your skin?	✓	
Are your pores clean and clear looking?		✓
Are your pores plugged or clogged?	✓	

Do your lips:	Never	Usually	Always
Chap only in winter?			✓
Chap at other times?			✓
Peel?		✓	
Show white spots?	✓		
Split, or crack at the corners?	✓		
Produce cold sores?	✓		
Does your lipstick bleed and edges smudge?	✓		

Goals: _____

_____

Date: _____

Your Wrinkle Questionnaire

Do you have:	Yes	No	
Horizontal lines in your forehead?		✓	
1 Vertical lines between eyebrows?	✓		74 ✓
2 Crow's-feet?	✓		86 ✓
Horizontal cheek lines?		✓	
Vertical cheek lines?		✓	
Vertical lines in front of your ears?	✓		
3 Nose-to-mouth lines?	✓		90 ✓
Lines over your lips?	✓		
Horizontal chin lines?		✓	
Sunburst lines from mouth over chin?		✓	
Center cheek hollows?		✓	
4 Jowls?	✓		104 ✓
5 Double chin?	✓		102
Drooping lips?		✓	
Drooping eyebrows?		✓	
Under-eye bags?	✓		84
Puffy eyelids?	✓		

Goals: _____ Date: _____

13

Your Facial Wrinkle Map

Defining your problems visually as well as verbally is a great help in overcoming them.

To define your wrinkles, you need a large piece of wax paper, or thin plastic, or a large clear plastic bag. You will use this to make a record of the problems to be eliminated. We find a large Baggie easiest to work with.

> With clear plastic tape, secure the *closed* bottom of the bag, if you're using one, to the upper part of the mirror of the medicine cabinet in your bathroom. The exact position will depend on your height. You should be able to see yourself clearly through the plastic.
>
> Using a cosmetic pencil such as eyebrow or lipstick pencil, or a grease pencil, outline your face on the plastic. Work downward from the top toward the bottom. Draw just the face, not the hair or neck and shoulder areas. Mark eyes, nose, ears.
>
> Mark your wrinkles on the plastic, matching what you see in the mirror. Remove the plastic from the mirror.
>
> Place a sheet of paper under the plastic, or inside if you are using a bag, to make it easier to see the markings. Choose the color that best suits your skin tone—peach, beige, or cream to brown.
>
> At the bottom of the plastic, or on the paper underneath, write down the specific wrinkles that will be your special targets, as, for example: ''Goals: Eradicate vertical wrinkles over nose, between brows. Get rid of crow's-feet. Eliminate nose to mouth wrinkles. Lose double chin.''
>
> Go through the facial exercises and ''smoothing'' techniques in this book and choose the exercises and smoothings that are designed to overcome the problems you have listed. Write down the page numbers below your list of ''Goals.''

Save your "facial map." You will be able to use this image over and over again, simply wiping way each wrinkle as you eliminate it.

Your Skin Care Questionnaire

This worksheet sets forth your beauty environment and your *present* beauty care techniques.

Climate: tropical _____ temperate __✓__ moist _____ dry _____

Air quality: clear __✓__ polluted _____ varies _____
    (country air)   (city air)

How often do you wash your face? ___*2 x / day*___

Do you rinse in hot water? __✓__ cool water? _____ tepid water? _____

What kind of cleaning agent do you use?
    soap __✓__ cream __✓__ other _____

What brand of soap or cleanser do you use? ___*always*___ *M. K.*

How long does it take to wash your face? ___*2 min.*___

How do you rinse your face? ___*yes*___

How does your face feel after washing?
    soft *MK* __✓__ greasy _____ tight __✓__ dry _____

How do you dry your face?
    terry towel __✓__ smooth towel _____ paper _____ air _____

Do you dry completely? ___*yes*___

Do you apply moisturizer to your face directly after washing? ___*yes*___

Is your face ever makeup-free and cream-free? ___*yes*___

What unguents (moisturizers, special creams, softeners, etc.) do you use?
___*MK Dubarry*___

How does your face feel immediately after you use that unguent? ___*soft*___

Do you use special cream or other substance to remove makeup? ___*MK soap*___

If yes, what kind or brand? ___*MK*___

If you apply a special cream around your eyes, describe it. ___*Dubarry*___

If yes, at night only? _____ Night and day? ___*yes*___

What other areas of your face receive special care? ___*eyes lines*___

Do you use a facial mask? ___*1 x / week*___

15

If yes, what kind? _MK_

How often? _1x/week_

Do you use a facial sauna? _no_

If yes, by yourself or professionally? _____ How often? _____

Do you steam your face? _no_

If yes, by yourself or professionally? _____ How often? _____

Do you massage your face? _no_

If yes, by yourself or professionally? _____ How often? _____

Are you *presently* doing any facial exercises? _no_

Goal: _____

Date: _____

Your Eye Care Questionnaire

	Yes	No
Is your vision 20/20?		✓
Do you wear glasses?	✓	
Do you wear contact lenses?		✓
If yes, what kind?		
Do you wear sunglasses?	✓	
If yes, do you wear them:		
Only in bright sunlight?		
All the time outdoors?	✓	
Outdoors and indoors?		✓
Do you exercise your eyes?		✓
If yes, do you exercise more than once a day?		✓
If you use eye cream or moisturizer, do you "fingerprint" it around your eye?		✓
If you wear eyeliner, do you take care not to stretch the eyelid while applying the liner?		✓
Do you use drops or eyewash in your eyes?	✓	
Do you work under eye-straining fluorescent lighting?	_work_	✓
Do you take care not to read or paint under poor light?	✓	

16

Do you take care not to rub your eyes with
the backs of your fists?

Do you think of your eye health in choosing
your meals?

Goals: _____

Date: _____

Your Foot Care Questionnaire

	Never	Usually	Always
Do your feet hurt?	✓		
Do you have bunions?	✓		
Did you ever have plantar warts on the soles of your feet?	✓		
Do you have calluses on the soles of your feet?	✓		
Do you have calluses on the rims of your heels? On your toes?	✓		
Do you have corns on your toes?	✓		
Have you ever visited a podiatrist?		✓	
Do you walk barefoot?		✓	
Do you change your shoes more than once a day?		✓	
Do you exercise your feet and ankles?	✓		
Do you swing your arms when you walk?		✓	
Do you try to walk daily, hands free of briefcase or shopping bag?	✓		
Did you ever have a professional pedicure?	✓		
Do you give yourself a pedicure?			✓
Do you buy shoes that hurt your feet?	✓		
Do you wear high heels (over 3 inches)?	✓		
Are you on your feet at least two hours every day?		✓	
Do you walk for exercise?	✓		
Do you walk more than one hour a day?	✓		

Do you run for exercise? _____ _____ _____

Do you actively exercise your feet and legs
more than 15 minutes a day? _____ _____ _____

Do you jog? _____ _____ _____

Do you jog more than 15 minutes a day? _____ _____ _____

Do you skip rope? _____ _____ _____

Do you cut your toenails straight across? _____ _____ _✓_

Do you have ingrown toenails? _____ _____ _____

Are your toes ever bluish in color? _____ _____ _____

Have you ever had a toe or foot infection? _____ _____ _____

Are there cracks or dry skin between your
toes? _____ _____ _____

Are your feet flat? __no__

Do you sometimes feel that your legs or feet are tired? __yes__

Do you fall often? __no__

Are your ankles weak? __no__

Goals: _____

_____

Date: _____

Part Two

GENERAL PREVENTION

Four

✄ALL ABOUT YOUR SKIN ✄

The skin is the largest organ in the body and is both a protector of the rest of the body and an eliminator of toxic wastes.

The skin of an average size person covers an area about 20 square feet and may represent as much as 15 percent of the total weight. If you are about 5 feet, 5 inches tall and weigh about 125 pounds, your skin is about 17 square feet in size and 19 pounds in weight. One square inch of skin contains some 19 million cells, 60 hairs that each grow from a separate follicle, 90 tiny oil glands, 19 feet of blood vessels, 650 sweat glands (except on the face and back, where there may be even more), and 19,000 sensory cells.

Skin thickness varies. The skin around your eyes and on your eyelids is very thin, about as thin as tissue paper. The skin on the heels of your feet, especially if you go barefoot or wear sandals, may be as thick as a quarter of an inch. The palms of your hands have much thicker skin than the back of your hands; this is one reason why the back of the hand appears to age much faster than the palm.

This elastic, flexible, soft, pliable, tough, durable covering called *skin*—through which one-third of your bloodstream flows—is wonderfully designed to protect your internal organs.

We're all familiar with the phrase about ''rubbing people the wrong way,'' or describing people as a ''soft touch,'' or ''to be handled with care'' or ''thick-skinned.'' When we irritate someone, we ''get under their skin.'' To be superficial about anything—knowledge or feeling—we often say, dismissingly, ''only skin deep.'' These metaphors are common because they bring familiar images to mind—our biggest organ, the mirror we hold to the world to examine our health, our personality, our personal habits.

21

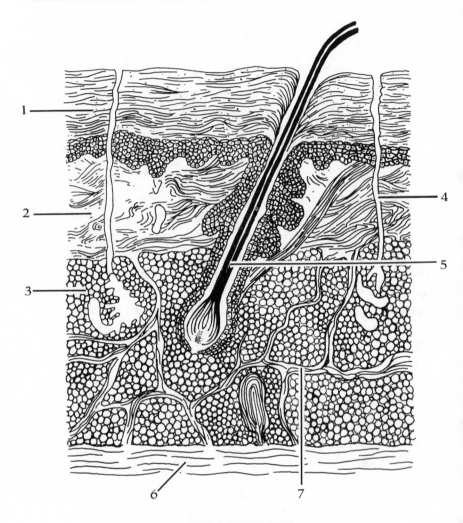

LAYERS OF THE SKIN

1. *Epidermis,* the outer layer of the skin that flakes off.
2. *Dermis,* the layer of the skin where the new cells grow.
3. *Fat* deposits that add softness to the skin.
4. *Sweat* ducts for perspiration.
5. *Hair* growing from hair follicles.
6. *Muscle* that controls the skin; the muscle tightens skin.
7. *Nerves* and nerve endings on surface of the skin.

The skin has more nerve terminals or endings that any other organ and is very sensitive. The nerve endings of your skin are constantly monitoring information about the outside world for use by the brain and adaptation by the body. The skin is continually regulating the temperature of the body. It keeps the organs inside the body at a constant, pleasant temperature, cooling you in summer and warming you in winter. One of the reasons that damage to the skin, such as a severe burn, is so serious is that body heat and fluids can be lost quickly without the protection of the skin.

When you are cold, the skin's nerves tell the brain. Result: the small blood vessels and capillaries that feed the skin shrink and tighten. The outer surface of the skin pulls together and "goose bumps" appear on your arms. This causes the hair on your arms, legs, and body to fluff up in an attempt to hold body heat near the skin. If the weather is very hot, the capillaries and blood supply near the surface of the skin dilate; more blood flows near the surface of the skin, the pores open, and perspiration, a natural body fluid, flows out and evaporates on the surface of the skin, making you feel cooler. Perspiration is mostly water—over 98 percent—plus a few salts and minerals from the body. If you are exercising or are otherwise physically active, your body might produce as much as two pints of perspiration in a day—a quart of liquid. Anxiety, nervousness, other emotional factors, an asthmatic or hypoglycemic attack, and certain other illnesses can cause you to sweat even when the atmosphere is cold—from the soles of your feet to your scalp.

ONE-THIRD OF YOUR BLOODSTREAM

The skin is a complex, seven-layered structure, but two of the layers are of primary importance: the dermis and the epidermis. The outer layer, called the *epidermis*, is actually a thin, multi-layered protein substance called *keratin*. Keratin is quite similar to the kind of cell that makes up your nails, as well as the antlers on deer, elk, cows, bulls and other horned animals.

Under the epidermis is the *dermis*, the layer that holds the sweat glands, the hair follicles, nerve endings, blood capillaries, oil glands, nerve tissue, and other elements, including fibroblasts, which, when you are under stress, can defend against intrusion of foreign matter. It is the dermis that contains the pigment that determines the actual color of the complexion. The number and size of blood vessels in the dermis cannot be seen through the upper layer of the skin, but when your blood vessels are free of debris and your circulation is good, you are aware of the bright red blood flowing through the dermis; your skin will have a flush and healthy glow. The reason your skin turns pink or even red when you are overheated or excited is that the activity, physical or mental, stimulates the blood flow. To have a healthy skin, you must keep the blood circulating well. Poor color, pallor, and a dull, sallow complexion almost inevitably indicate poor circulation.

To help keep the skin elastic, avoid stretching it and misusing it by pulling, nervous fingering, or careless rubbing. The greatest detriment to skin flexibility, however, is sun abuse. Exposure to the sun increases concentration of the color agent in the skin. Overexposure thickens, hardens, and dries the epidermis and shrinks the dermis. Several bad sunburns can do lifelong damage to the skin.

When the skin is cut, bruised, or otherwise damaged, the process of healing starts immediately. Blood flows to clean the opening; then it coagulates and the vessels contract to prevent the entry of bacteria and foreign matter. The clotting blood forms fine threadlike links that weave together to join the sides of the wound.

Within 24 hours after the bleeding, any foreign material or bacteria normally will be attacked, broken down, and absorbed by white blood cells. At the same time, the thick epidermal cells begin to divide and multiply. The outer surface becomes hard, and a scab forms over the wound. Under that scab, the sides of the wound join and the skin is reformed. It takes about a week to reconstitute the dermis, and less than a month for the upper layer to be completely normal again.

When the bacteria or other foreign matter attacking the skin opening is too lethal for the white blood cells to handle, infection occurs. Infections cause formation of pus, which is a collection of dead white cells and bacteria. This pus presses against nerves of healthy skin tissue and causes pain. If the infected matter gets into the blood, it can be carried to other parts of the body and other organs. Dead skin and pus can sometimes be seen as part of a boil or pimple.

Skin troubles, including blackheads and whiteheads, have a variety of causes, such as overactive glands putting too much oil into the small pores of the skin. Wrinkled skin comes in part from too *little* moisture. Some people suffer from both problems. Surprisingly, however, the two problems can be treated similarly.

Skin health depends largely on the vitality of the blood flow. Thus, both acne and wrinkled skin can be helped by exercise and other forms of stimulation of the blood flow, from proper cleansing and moisturizing of the skin, and from a diet that provides the nutrients the body needs to stimulate cell growth from the ''basement membrane,'' which is a thin, flexible separation between the protective epidermis and the dermis.

The cells in your skin actually form far below the skin and move slowly to the surface layer. Normally, cells generated on the bottom level of the epidermis make their way to the skin surface in a little over fifteen days. When they reach the surface, they are old, thin, and scalelike. These old cells, dull and flaky in appearance, need to be washed off and/or rubbed away. With them they carry grime, dirt, pollution, body wastes, and bacteria.

As you grow older, your cells do not replenish themselves as quickly or as vigorously as they did in early years. Sometimes the cells do not flake away, the growing cells do not dislodge them, and the cleansing which is an aid to nature does not do the job, either. Then it is necessary to help nature—by brushing and scrubbing away these dead cells to reveal the new growth beneath. This rubbing is called *epider-abrasion*. Epider-abrasion is necessary to help remove the old, dead, dry, flaky cells and make way for the new growth. It simply aids nature. Since the older skin is often thin, the practice exposes the new cells quickly, in turn encouraging new growth of cells, and thus actually slowing down the aging process while making you look more beautiful at the same time.

When the graying film of old cells, dirt, and stale makeup are gone, your complexion will be livelier and more translucent. It will also feel smoother and more moist and will look younger.

Black women often complain of an ''ashy'' look to their skins. That comes from these dead, gray—ashy—cells lying on top of the dark underskin. If you look at skin under a magnifying glass, you usually can see these tiny flaky dead cells.

Not only your face, but also your body needs to be freed of all the old dead cells. The skin on your elbows, heels, toes, knees, and buttocks seem to require help, i.e., brushing, the most. However, all the skin on your body, even your back and shoulders as well as your stomach, breasts, and arms, should be rubbed, brushed, or buffed in some way every single day.

Buffing and brushing the skin is usually thought of as a way of unplugging blocked oil ducts and as a treatment for acne and other oily skin problems. But is is just as helpful for the older skin. Most older people believe that brushing will dry their skin. Actually the effect is exactly the opposite. Because it gets rid of the upper layer of the skin, stimulates oil flow and new cell growth, and opens the layers of the skin, it enables the nourishment you put on your skin, in the form of moisturizers and creams, to work more effectively.

Skin ''throws off'' dead skin on the upper layer every four hours. It is the dead skin lying on the surface of the skin, combined with oils and other body wastes and atmospheric pollution, that makes your face dirty. Cleaning your face several times a day is first aid for lifelong skin beauty.

IS THERE A BEST WAY TO CLEANSE THE SKIN?

This is a question every woman is likely to ask. While we recommend soap and water, health, age, environment, custom, and climate all can be factors in choosing a cleansing method. Some people believe that we bathe too often in the United States! Others, including nature-oriented physicians, insist a daily bath or shower is essential. Doctors on the other side of the fence suggest we should wash our hair and skins less often as we gain years. The authors, after extensive research leading to the finding that the skin feels, looks, and is softer when it is washed often, belong to the pro-washing school.

Soap is one of the inventions that changed the world. The

26

advent of soap cut down on infection and did more to diminish disease than any other cause. It was invented during the third century A.D. in several different places in the world, including China, India, and Europe. Soap is, today, still the main cleansing agent for the skin.

There is a great difference among soaps. The kind or brand you choose should be dictated by your skin. Soap is usually identified as ''dry skin'' or ''oily skin'' soap. Dry skin soap has more oil in it and is usually bland, white, and nonirritating. Oily skin soap may include additional ingredients such as seaweed, oatmeal, or other vegetable products. Brown and bumpy looking soap is often used for oily skin; clear amber soap is sometimes used for dry skin.

There are acne soaps and deodorant soaps, perfumed soaps and nonperfumed soaps. Some soaps, notably perfumed ones, can cause allergic reactions. Choosing a soap that's best for you often can be simply a case of trial and error, until you find one that cleans and does no damage.

Many people think they are allergic to soap. It's more likely they are allergic to a particular ingredient—often the perfume. Allergists and dermatologists tell us that their patients benefit from the use of a number of nonperfumed, bland soaps.

The more you wash your face, the cleaner it is and the clearer your complexion will be. Washing your face every four or five hours, rinsing carefully, and lubricating can do a lot for your skin if you are in a dirty atmosphere. Morning and night can be adequate if you live in a clean, dry area.

Every soap produces an alkaline reaction. Since the normal acid mantle of the skin is protection against infection, some women like to add a *tiny* amount of apple cider vinegar or lemon juice to the final rinse water.

Always rinse away *every trace* of soap, and rinse quite a bit longer even after you think you've rid your face of it. Remember that it is not so much the type of soap that's used but how thoroughly it's rinsed away that makes the difference in the skin's clarity, tone, and any feeling of ''dryness.'' A feeling of dryness or tightness usually indicates that more rinsing is needed.

Here are some general rules for cleansing with soap:
1. Avoid scrubbing with any soaps—unless your doctor has ordered a specific technique.
2. Avoid very hot water. Warm for the body, very warm for the face, is a good general choice, although hot and cold water have their own special benefits too—for instance on your feet and legs to stimulate the circulation.
3. Don't use deodorant or medicated soap unless advised to do so by your physician.

The skin needs hydration—from the outside by washing, and from the inside by the drinking water. Eight glasses of water daily should be basic. Not drinking enough water encourages wrinkles.

We recommend that you wash your face with soap twice a day and with plain water much oftener—as much as you can. Ten washings will only benefit your skin! Try washing your face ten times a day and you'll see. In ten days, you'll be astonished, we believe, at the improved color, tone, and clarity of your skin.

While our research doesn't indicate soap dries the skin at all if it is well rinsed, if your skin is very dry some of you may want to alternate soap and water cleansing with a cream or gel cleansing.

CLEANSING CREAMS, CLEANSING LOTIONS, OILS AND GELS

Cleansing cream was already in use in Rome two thousand years ago. Today, the most popular skin cleanser is cold cream. Most cleansing creams melt on the skin. In the jar their temperature is about 70°F., but when put on the skin, with its 98° temperature, they liquify and form a slick surface. When the surface is wiped, waste— soil, makeup, dead cells, and other debris—is cleaned from the skin.

Oils can be used for lubricating as well as for cleansing. Any vegetable oil—corn oil, peanut oil, or safflower oil—is an excellent cleanser. Baby oil and mineral oil are to be avoided—baby oil because it contains mineral oil. While mineral oil and baby oil may seem, initially, to be beneficial to the skin, in actual fact mineral oil leaches

28

natural oil from the skin so that, after prolonged use, a woman suddenly finds her face wrinkled and often itchy. Thinking that her skin's need is for oil, she piles on more mineral oil or a mineral oil-based product, and only aggravates the condition. Astonishingly, some women who think they have excessively dry skin because of the wrinkles and/or itchiness actually have oily skin.

Generally it's thought that it's lack of oil that makes a skin dry. The truth is that the skin becomes dry if it lacks water—moisture. The natural oils of the skin emulsify and help to bind the water, encouraging the skin to be pliant and supple.

REMOVING THE CREAMS AND OILS

Usually tissue is used to wipe off the cream, oil, or gel; but tissue, it should be remembered, is made from wood, and even fine tissue can leave microscopic splinters on the skin, so think twice about using it. Instead, use disposable cotton balls or swatches of absorbent cotton. You can use cheesecloth, too, but that requires washing after each use and few modern women want to be bothered with that chore.

The very best way to wash your face is perhaps the simplest. Use your fingertips only, and plain clear water, warm water. You will find that most cream will liquify and easily wash away at about 110°F. And most household water is about 150°F. directly from the faucet. Here is a step by step procedure that will ensure the proper cleansing of your face:

Wash hands carefully.
Leave warm water faucet running.
Apply soap to the face, directly from the bar—just gently stroke the cake across your face.
Using wet hand, work up lather on your face.
Soap the nose and chin area carefully.
Avoid the eye area.
Soap and lather neck.
Rinse the face and neck with very warm water.
Rinse twice as long as you think is necessary.
Dry face and neck carefully with a terry towel.

Ernesto Lazlo, the famous beauty and cosmetics counselor who is a consultant for socialites and movie stars, recommends very hot water and between thirty and fifty rinsings. He tells his patient-clients to use nothing but their fingertips. He stresses the natural beauty of good, clear, and healthy skin.

Unless advised to because of a specific problem, don't put ice on your face. The skin is too delicate for application of ice cubes. (For exceptions, see the sections on Skin Problems later in this chapter.)

If you do use tissue, either out of habit or for convenience, do not drag or rub the tissue across your face. Press the tissue on your face and pull off the top layer, then gently wipe and blot the skin with the lower layer.

The most expensive cosmetics and the most carefully formulated unguents and moisturizers cannot make a poor skin look beautiful. Keeping your skin clean and clear is basic to beauty, but it takes time. Coverings are just camouflage and really do not help. Your makeup can look only as lovely as the skin beneath it. That is why we recommend a program that is suited and fashioned by you, just for your skin, one that emphasizes cleansing, combined with exfoliating —dermabrasion of a sort.

SKIN PEELERS

Every once is a while you'll notice ads about skin peelers or other abrasives that will rid the skin of small wrinkles. These products or treatments, chemically or mechanically, take off the upper epidermis layer—and sometimes part of the lower dermis layer too.

The concept behind the "skin peeler" is that the skin will replenish itself with new skin that is less wrinkled and smoother. There is more than one kind of commercial peeler. One type contains chemicals that strip the skin. These we don't recommend. In another type, the "peeling agent" comes from the acids of fruits. It is gentle in action yet effective. You can use it weekly with benefit. You'll be astonished to see the dry skin that will come off, and delighted by the refreshed and glowing look of your skin.

As we have emphasized before, daily washing is important to exfoliating (sloughing off) the dead skin. Dry brushing aids, too.

However, use only natural products for brushing. Plastic or nylon products can cause tiny breaks in the skin. There are a variety of natural bristle complexion brushes available for your face, and loofah or other natural "brushers" for the body. Your entire body should be washed at least once a day, and more often in summer or if you are involved in work that causes excessive perspiration.

SKIN PROBLEMS

Many suffer from annoying and chronic skin problems which aggravate the worry about wrinkles or the potential of wrinkles. Acne, bacteria infections such as impetigo and cellulitis, scabies, dermatilis, and psoriasis as well as warts should be treated by a doctor who has special training in recognizing and alleviating the unpleasant symptoms.

AIR TRAVEL

A very modern cause of premature wrinkling is constant air travel. You can handle this problem—once you're aware of it. The atmosphere in a high-flying jet-liner is very drying to the skin. Before and during flights, wise women, and men too, will bathe their faces well with very light moisturizers and renew the moisturizer if the flight lasts more than two hours. While in an airplane, it is best to eat lightly if at all, avoid alcohol, and drink lots of water.

SUN

While the sun is *essential* to life and health and to the growth of the food we eat, more and more it is recognized that it can be extremely damaging to the skin and can be a particular cause of premature wrinkling.

Exposure to the ultraviolet rays of the sun produces an increased concentration of *melanin*, the coloring agent of the skin. In fair-skinned people this increase in melanin produces tanning. Freckles result from special concentrations of melanin. When the melanin increases evenly, a suntan results. While providing a feeling of warmth and well-being, and while seeming to help some skin conditions such as psoriasis and acne, the sun can have disastrous after-effects.

If you are untanned and spend several hours exposed to tropical sun, the protective oils of your skin will be overtaxed and the resultant painful sunburn can do serious and permanent damage to your skin. Women who constantly sunbathe without using suntan oils or a sun block often look leathery in time. ''Outdoors'' Western women often show this effect. This is because the upper levels of their skin actually become annealed to the dermis layer.

The weathered cowboy look sometimes is only part of the damage. Cancer of the skin is more prevalent in people who are constantly in the sun. Sailors, farmers, and construction workers are more prone to the disease than the general population.

These warnings about the perils of the sun don't mean that the sun doesn't benefit. The key is to take it easy. Get used to it gradually. Avoid sunburns. Avoid the combination of sun-windburn. Use a moisturizer on your skin when you're outdoors for long, and a sun block that really works. Some of the most highly advertised are worthless.

Wear a hat! Some people with very fair, very fine skin, like red-headed actress-beauty expert Arlene Dahl, should never appear outdoors in the sunshine without a hat or parasol to shade the face. Arlene doesn't.

Enjoy the sun. Benefit from it. But treat it with respect. Be a sun worshipper in the sense of the ancients, who daily gave thanks to the sun and carried their sick to mountain and hilltops and exposed them to the health-giving rays of the sun. But they didn't remain there to bake as many moderns do on summer beaches.

Remember Kipling's line: ''Only mad dogs and Englismen go out in the mid-day sun.'' If you must sunbathe, avoid the sun at least between 11 A.M. and 3 P.M.

ALCOHOL ABUSE

Alcohol, like the sun, is also misunderstood. Overconsumption can cause the appearance of tiny red veins around the nose, and often eventually the bulbous ''whiskey nose'' that became the trademark of the great entertainer, W. C. Fields. Overconsumption also leads to dehydration, which encourages wrinkles.

But, contrary to what is often thought, *moderate* drinking does not adversely affect the skin, nor shorten life. Research by the Human Population Laboratory in California brought the report that "those who never drank did not differ significantly from those who drank moderately."

Another study showed that those who drank moderately lived longer than abstainers, and both live much longer than alcoholics, but there are some conditions, such as hypoglycemia, which call for abstention from any alcohol, or, at the most, a rare drink. A famous TV talk show personality recently said that a single glass of wine could cause him a sleepless night.

However, for some people, particularly when they pass the 70 mark, some doctors recommend an occasional, or daily, highball or glass of beer or wine. It is important to keep in mind that a glass of table wine, a bottle of beer, and a highball—with 1½ ounces of spirits—are about equivalent in alcoholic content. The calories vary: 105 calories for 1½ ounces of gin, vodka, rum, or whiskey; 101 calories for 8 ounces of beer; 87 calories for 3½ ounces of table wine; 141 calories for 3½ fluid ounces of dessert wine.

For a large-pored, W. C. Fields' nose, dermatologists have few solutions. With such cases we have recommended frequent washing of the face with soap and water, two times daily with soap and several more times with plain water, followed by an "ice toner." The nose should be gently massaged with an ice cube wrapped in a piece of thin cotton. After the ice bath, let the nose become partly dry from the atmosphere and then nourish it (and the rest of the face) with a moisturizer.

A facial mask three times weekly is also recommended for this condition. This treatment, combined with a diet rich in beauty foods free of heavy spices, often helps improve the condition. Prevention is the better way. Moderation and balance are essential to health and are the keys to enjoyment of alcoholic beverages, too.

BROKEN VEINS

Broken veins from bruises or broken blood vessels can be removed by most dermatologists. These broken blood vessels can result from too hot or too cold water being used on the face. Avoid ice or ice water on your face or any other place on your body. The drastic change in temperature will trap blood inside a small vessel and can cause the vessels to burst, forming a broken vein.

Tiny broken veins around the nose can result from use of overly hot water on the skin, or perhaps from too close exposure while giving yourself a steam facial—putting your head under a towel while you steam yourself over boiling water. Sometimes the problem can result from setting the heat too high on an electric facial sauna. If you have broken veins, facial saunas and steam saunas are best avoided.

STRESS

Stress is a worse enemy for your skin than the sun. There is no life without some stress; stress is the fuel that gets you moving, to do almost anything. But too much stress can cause terrible problems, from skin rash and wrinkles to a heart attack.

Stress can cause acne, sweat retention, bruises, and some doctors believe hives also are stress-induced, as well as allergic manifestations.

There are rashes of stress origins that cause a tingling of the skin, prompting a person to scratch, thus aggravating the itch, which in turn aggravates the rash. Itching is a common reaction to excess stress. A doctor wise in the way of people will prescribe an anti-itch topical medication. (Sometimes ''itches'' and even blisters which are identified as ''stress reactions'' are actually allergies; and if you suspect you need an allergist, choose someone who is *up-to-date* on theories and research about *causes*, which often can be the additives in products.)

Tension and stress set the face into unattractive patterns, a fact that can cause friends and even relatives to feel like running! Unfortunately, few of us are so compassionate as to seek those whose manner is vexed and anxious or who appear unhappy. Inability to handle stress must be listed as an enemy of beauty—and of a smooth skin.

Meditation can help, as well as prayer. You can help handle stress simply by saying twenty times a day the phrase made famous in the Twenties: "Every day in every way, I'm getting better and better!" It really works.

WARTS

Warts are small, nonmalignant tumors of the skin, and topical application of castor oil can free you from them, whether they occur on hands, feet, or elsewhere on the body. Ascorbic acid powder is credited with clearing up seed or plantar warts within a week. If these remedies don't work, consult a doctor. Warts should not be "frozen," cut away, or removed chemically except by a doctor.

MOLES

Moles are raised brown marks that appear as blemishes on the skin. As skin ages, these often become more prevalent and change shape. They are sometimes thought to be liver spots, a scattering of dark patches of skin resembling large freckles which are caused by a collection of melanin but can become malignant. Medical help should always be sought if any increase in size or shape, number or color is noticed. If hair grows from a mole that is on your face or some other visible part of your body, do not pluck the hair with a tweezer. It is better to carefully trim the hair with a small sharp manicure scissors.

STRETCH MARKS

While many experts claim there is little that present medical or even folklore knowledge can do about these light-colored tracks that mark the tummy, lower abdomen, thighs, buttocks, or other parts of the body, others claim they can be eradicated. Almost everyone has them; everyone who has them hates them.

The stretch marks are technically called *striae*, which means channels or furrows. They are usually associated with distensions of the skin, such as those caused by yo-yo weight gains and losses.

Striae gravidarum, a term from the Latin, refers to the marks that come from pregnancy. However, they are just as common in the thighs, usually of people who have never been pregnant. Fewer men than women suffer from striae. It is believed that striae form when the skin is stretched beyond its flexibility.

When the underlying elastic proteins of the skin break down because of stretching, the upper skin or epidermis becomes detached from the fibrous collagen tissue, which is the elastic protein that keeps the skin together. Thus, striae appear.

If you are pregnant, or very thin and planning to gain weight, or overweight and planning to lose weight, a program of care will help you avoid stretch marks. The traditional method is to rub the enlarging area with cocoa butter, but that always makes the subject smell like cocoa. Vitamin E has been used with reported good results. A capsule of vitamin E will provide just about the right amount for an application. Rub the oily substance into the stretch marks just before bedtime, or after a bath when your skin might be most receptive to absorbing the oils. Continue to use the vitamin E compound until you are sure that there is no further danger of developing the nasty little tracks.

If you already are a victim of the light-colored ribbon marks, you can submit to surgery, a drastic solution which we do not recommend unless you have a special need, such as being an entertainer or professional model where the marks could interfere with your career.

Some people bleach the areas where the stretch marks occur. To do this, use a soothing bleach cream, such as Mitchums, Artra, or one of the many light bleach creams that some black women use to unify the color on their faces or hands. Make sure these bleach creams do not contain any mercury, a dangerous product that can be absorbed into the skin. Any bleach used should have a moisturizing, nondrying base.

Rub the cream into your skin every night, and in about six weeks the bleaching will make the marks less noticeable. This is particularly true of stretch marks on the side of the breast that are due to engorgement during pregnancy or lactation. If you use the bleach on your breasts, support the breast with one hand while you rub in the cream with the other. It would be unfortunate to break the delicate tissue further while trying to improve it.

Another method is to cream and then lightly rub with a very soft cosmetic brush or stiff terry washcloth. This helps the skin to renew itself; it is thought that new skin may not show the stretch marks so much.

Luci Flint, the beauty authority who is the foremost expert on the aloe vera plant, declares that massage with cream truly rich in aloe vera will put an end to these tracks that mark the skin. Mentioned seven times in the Bible, aloe vera was carried into battle by ancient Egyptians, who put aloe vera leaves on wounds to heal them. Aloe vera is now being used in a number of hospitals, to encourage new skin growth after surgery and also to heal burns. In Mexico and Jamaica, aloe vera leaves are used to heal or prevent sunburn. Luci Flint recommends use of aloe vera cream throughout pregnancy and for several months after to prevent stretch marks, and she insists faithful massage with the cream will eradicate them too.

DRUGS AND WRINKLES

Tranquilizers such as Valium and Librium, tobacco and marijuana, diet pills with amphetamines, as well as overuse of alcohol, coffee, and other drugs, including antibiotics, can be very detrimental to your skin. Starved skin is dull, lifeless, and unattractive. The skin of a drug addict soon becomes drab and wrinkled. A person who becomes an addict at 18 can look like an old man or woman at 25—and be dead soon after.

Drugs produce a dulling effect or an unreal feeling of well-being. Both of these effects can and do help people deal with temporarily difficult situations, but cannot solve long-term problems. Amphetamines, sometimes called ''pep pills,'' keep the body ready for action with the muscles tense and the heart and blood flow rate up. People who use the drug often enjoy excitement and hyperactivity—but are victims of trembling, dizziness, and insomnia; many become dependent on them. The pep pills temporarily curb appetite. Besides the harm of the drugs themselves, your skin is further injured because often the user forgets to eat the nutrient-rich food vital for good health and good skin. Nervous energy replaces natural energy. Further, the drug may be addictive.

The most frequently used drug is probably caffeine, a stimulant which affects the central nervous system. Caffeine is found in cola drinks and tea as well as coffee and chocolate. It would take large quantities of caffeine to really hurt you, but if you drink coffee and cola and eat chocolate, in addition to taking headache and cold pills which may also contain caffeine, you are inviting trouble.

Depression, fatigue, and a feeling of dullness are often experienced when you attempt to cut down on your intake of coffee or caffeine in general. The solution is to take a drink of fresh fruit or vegetable juice—a healthful pickup that aids your skin too.

SKIN HAZARDS

Just as injudicious exposure to the sun can cause skin problems, so can overexposure to other elements of the environment, such as wind, severe cold, steam heat, air conditioning, and pollution. All these can dry the skin. To counteract them, keep the heat and air conditioning as low as possible, clean your face often, and keep your skin well moisturized.

Chlorine-treated water is drying, too. The solution: shower as soon as possible after being in a pool and keep your skin well moisturized with products that really penetrate the skin, such as those containing substantial amounts of aloe vera and avocado oil, and possibly further enriched by A, E, and B vitamins.

DIET

Faulty Diet: Of course not all of you will want to change your eating habits so radically as to eat *only* those foods that are good for your skin. (Few of us want to do that.) Each of us came into the world with our own, unique taste-buds and taste consciousness, but under the tutelage of parents, grandparents, or peers we rapidly learn that some foods are considered good and we learn to dislike others, and many of us came to equate sweet foods with good times and rewards. The important thing to keep in mind, however, is that certain foods benefit your skin, and that you should seek to incorporate them into your diet as much as possible. Too often we eat the foods that do us, and our skins, little or no good and we have no appetite left for what will help us toward our goal of being beautiful.

Foods to Avoid: The foods that we might do well to avoid are those with ''empty'' calories: pies, cakes, pastries, ice cream, ''fluffy'' white bread, and sugar-rich foods generally, including many prepared cereals, and soft drinks.

Foods to Favor—ABC's for Skin Beauty: A sound and varied diet is essential to a lovely skin and to prevention and reversal of wrinkles. The number one requirement of the skin is protein, which is essential to cell building. It is found in complete form in meat, fish, poultry, eggs, and dairy products, and in incomplete form in nuts, grains, vegetables, and to small degree in some fruits.

Foods rich in vitamins are also important to skin beauty, particularly those high in vitamins A (often called the ''beauty vitamin''), C, B_2, E, and F. Recent research indicates that pantothenic acid, commonly known in the cosmetic world as panthenol, and para-aminobenzoic acid (PABA) are important too. So are nucleic acids and an array of minerals, particularly iron, sulfur, calcium, silicon, sodium, chlorine, and zinc.

Some of the foods that are beneficial to the skin are the following:

A - abalone, alfalfa (leaves, sprouts), almonds, anchovies, apples, apricots, artichokes (globe and Jerusalem or American), asparagus, avocados

B - bamboo shoots, bananas, barley, bass, bean sprouts, beef (lean), beets and beet greens, blackberries, blueberries, bluefish, brains, Brazil nuts, broccoli, Brussels sprouts, buckwheat, butter, buttermilk

C - cabbage, carrots, cauliflower, celery, cheese, cherries, chicken, chives, citrus fruits, corn, crab, cranberries, cucumbers, currants

D - dandelion greens, dates (included to induce sleep)

E - eggplant, eggs, endives

F - fennel, figs, fish, frogs legs, all kinds of fresh and dried fruits, fruit juices

G - garlic in foods, or chopped fine and placed on the back of the tongue and swallowed with water, or in capsules (besides being good for skin and other organs, it helps reduce blood pressure), gooseberries, grapes, green beans, green leafy vegetables, guava (fresh)

H - halibut, herring, honey

K - kale, kefir, kidney, kiwi fruit

L - lamb, leeks, lentils, lettuce, lima beans, liver

M - mangos (fresh), melon, milk (especially whole), millet, molasses (blackstrap), mushrooms, mustard greens

N - nasturtium leaves, nectarines, nuts

O - oatmeal, oils (unsaturated, such as safflower, sesame, sunflower, and corn), onions, oysters

P - papaya, parsley, parsnips, peaches, peanuts, pears, peas, peppers (green and red), persimmons, pimiento, plantains, plums, pork, potatoes (white and sweet), poultry, prunes

R - radishes, raisins, raspberries, rhubarb, rice (particularly brown), rutabagas

S - salmon (fresh, canned, too, though it is very high in sodium), sardines, scallops, seafood, sesame seeds, butter and oil), shallots, shrimp, soybeans (including sprouts and flour), spinach, squash, strawberries, sunflower seeds (an especially good source of D, E, and B complex vitamins, as well as minerals and unsaturated oils and fatty acids), Swiss chard, swordfish

T - tomatoes, tuna, turkey, turnips (including greens—rich in vitamins A and C and calcium, iodine, iron, and other minerals)

V - veal, vegetables of all kinds, raw and cooked

W - walnuts, watercress, watermelon, wheat germ

Y - yams, yeast (brewer's, kefir), yogurt

Z - zucchini

Five

🌿ALL ABOUT YOUR EYES🌿

"Laugh lines" can appear at the corners of the eyes of a person as young as the early twenties, deepening into crow's-feet during the thirties, particularly when the person smokes. No one yet has looked into why smoking encourages crow's-feet; it's known only that it does. Each cigarette uses up 25 mg. of vitamin C, a fact that may be associated with crow's-feet. For this reason, smokers should make sure their daily diet is high in foods rich in vitamin C; for this reason, some imaginative companies have begun to market a special vitamin C-based tablet specifically for smokers.

Your eyes need all the help they can get. There are very few people who have perfect eyesight. An astonishing number of young people wear glasses or contact lens. Better doctors, frequent and more extensive examinations may be the reasons; or poor nutrition, as well as inadequate lighting.

Dr. John Ott, a retired banker, has spent most of his adult life researching light—first as a hobby and then as a dedicated full-time occupation. Dr. Ott declares that light entering the eyes influences the endocrine system, which in turn influences the production and release of hormones for the control of body chemistry. His research showed that the chemistry of the cells in plants and animals could be influenced by the interaction of the different wavelengths of light. Pink fluorescent lights have been shown to be particularly harmful, affecting personality as well as health and being particularly conducive to quarrelsomeness and tension. Dr. Ott's Environmental Health and Light Research Institute in Sarasota, Florida, has supported several studies at medical schools which demonstrated that when certain wavelengths are missing, such as the ultraviolet, photosynthesis is incomplete and an unbalanced chemical response results. Without the ultraviolet segment of the spectrum in particular, the normal process of mitosis or cell division does not take place.

If we lived truly naturally, we would depend only on the light of day. All artificial lighting represents some sort of distortion from natural day or sunlight. Window glass, automobile glass, and the usual eyeglasses filter out the important ultraviolet rays of the spectrum. Dr. Ott urges ''full spectrum'' eyeglasses and sunglasses for eye health and for general health too.

This too-brief report of Dr. Ott's fascinating contributions is pertinent here because any time normal cell division fails to take place, wrinkles are encouraged; whenever anyone is exposed to inadequate lighting, there is eyestrain, which in turn leads to tension wrinkles. So make sure your lighting is the best possible, investigate full-spectrum lighting, and whenever you can, wear full-spectrum glasses outdoors. If you are going to be spending long hours on ski slopes or on the sea, try to find full-spectrum tinted glasses so that the sun reflecting on snow and sea won't cause you to squint—and wrinkle.

Eye muscles should be exercised. Since the skin around the eyes is very fine and delicate, exercising must be done with care, using fingertip pressure only. Never drag the fingers over the skin. That could cause stretching and wrinkling. The fingers should always be picked up from one point and put down at another, never allowed to slide or drag. When applying eye makeup, take care not to stretch the skin. Regarding eye makeup, be particularly diligent about keeping the makeup contamination free. Never moisten mascara with saliva! Some authorities recommend that you discard mascara after three months simply to reduce any risk of contamination.

Don't overdo when you exercise your eyes. It is best to exercise them for half a minute or less three times a day. You'll find it relaxing, too. Exercises for the eyes are included in the exercise section.

By doing no more than the practical preventive action of seeing your opthamologist (eye physician) or optometrist (doctor of optometry) once every year or two, most people can expect to have fairly good vision to a very old age. If diagnosed early, many serious eye conditions can be prevented, corrected, or treated.

Foods to Favor—ABC's for Eye Health: The route to eye health and simultaneous prevention or reversal of wrinkles is fourfold: good illumination, adequate relaxation, exercises plus ''smoothings,'' and, of course, good nutrition. Here are the ABC's for eye health; the foods you should favor include the following:

A - apricots, asparagus, avocados

B - barley, beef, beet greens, blackberries, Brussels sprouts, butter

C - cabbage, carrots, cauliflower, cheese, corn, cucumbers

D - duck

E - eel, egg yolk, endives

F - fennel, figs

G - gooseberries

H - halibut

K - kumquats (fresh)

L - leafy vegetables, including lettuce; liver, loganberries

M - milk (whole), mustard greens

N - nasturtium leaves, nectarines, most nuts

O - oats, onions, oranges, organ meats, oysters

P - papaya, parsley, parsnips, peaches, pears, peas (green), peppers (green and red), pimiento, plums, poultry

R - radishes, raspberries, rhubarb

S - strawberries, sweet potatoes, Swiss chard

T - tomatoes

W - watercress, winter squash

Y - yeast (brewer's, kefir)

Six

TEETH AND WRINKLES

The state of health of your teeth has a direct relationship to wrinkles. If you have any kind of tooth problem, you have stress, a basic cause of premature wrinkling.

Teeth are hard, durable, bonelike combinations of enamel, dentine, and inner pulp. Their function is to help prepare food for digestion and to make the sounds of speech clearer. If even one tooth is lost, one or more wrinkles is encouraged.

The most common disease in the United States is not the common cold, it is tooth decay. One out of five persons has lost his or her teeth by age 40; 90 percent of American men, women, and children have a dental problem. Soft, sweet, and sticky food does not cause tooth decay, it only encourages it. Bacteria in the mouth, which feed on the carbohydrates in the sugary food, attack the tooth enamel and gradually form a small weakness. This enlarges to form a cavity. The result can be a variety of dental problems, not only toothaches, but abscesses. Gum infection is a frequent result, and from that teeth are likely to loosen and may have to be extracted. The loss of teeth is a major cause of wrinkles around the mouth, chin, and even cheeks. If tooth loss is followed by ill-fitting dentures, wrinkling is further encouraged; chewing may become difficult so that changes are made to a ''softer'' diet, which encourages poor elimination, which in turn encourages poor skin and more wrinkles.

From infancy on, everyone should be taught to give his or her teeth the best possible care so that the ''permanent teeth,'' which start coming in usually at age 5, will, like the heart, last a lifetime.

When permanent teeth are lost, they should be replaced immediately by false teeth. Ideally, dentures or ''false teeth'' should be an exact duplicate of the teeth they replace. The dentures should be checked by the dentist at least once a year, just as normal teeth are, to make sure the fit is tight but comfortable. Poorly fitted false teeth almost inevitably lead to tiny losses of the jawbone, encouraging wrinkles. If a tooth is lost from a denture it should be replaced as quickly as possible, and care should be taken that they fit perfectly, otherwise wrinkles related to the loss will appear in a matter of weeks.

Most of us were taught to brush twice a day. Brushing after every meal is better. After eating certain foods, blackstrap molasses or grapefruit, for instance, it's imperative. Both attack the enamel. It you can't clean your teeth after eating either of those items, forego them. If that's not possible, then eat some celery or an apple or other natural tooth cleansers.

Use a natural bristle brush and clean up and down, never across. Brush your gums too. If bleeding occurs, this indicates the possibility of a vitamin C deficiency. Use dental floss at least nightly to remove food particles between your teeth and near the gum line. Twice daily is better. Daily massage of the gums by thumb and forefinger is recommended.

Faulty bite is a common problem which can lead to premature wrinkling and a variety of disorders, including hearing loss, asthma, and nervousness. Because of the recently recognized importance of the bite in dental and overall health, the American Equilibration Society was formed by dentists and physicians, on an international basis, to study, prevent, and treat the symptoms of a dysfunction of the joints that connect the lower jaw to the skull. The usual correction is achieved by fitting one or more teeth, or even the entire lower jaw, with a natural-color ''splint'' to correct under or overbite. Clinicians report that correcting rough and overclosed dental occlusions benefits hearing and equilibrium, frees patients from pain about the teeth, face, head, and temporomandibular joints, and relieves patients suffering from dizziness or vertigo. Sometimes the improvements occur instantly with the mere fitting of the splint. Wrinkles can be diminished so radically by implacement of the splint that there seems to be an ''instant face life.''

Foods to Avoid: Unwise between-meal snacking is the principal source of most of the sweet, nutritionally poor foods we eat. It will take a little planning in the beginning to change snack habits, but before long you will find that nutritious between-meal snacks are decidedly more delicious as well as far better for your teeth.

The foods to avoid are those low in nutrients and high in sugar, including: sugar itself, honey, jams, jellies; baked sweet goods; chocolate bars, candies, lozenges, regular gum, and regular soft drinks.

Foods to Favor—ABC's for Tooth Health: All vitamin-rich foods, especially those containing vitamins A, C, and D, will help your teeth last your lifetime. Calcium, silicon, chlorine, and fluorine from natural sources are important for healthy teeth. In general, the goal should be to favor foods high in nutritional value and low in sugar, at meal-time or for between-meal snacking.

A - abalone, alfalfa sprouts

B - beets, broccoli, Brussels sprouts

C - carp, cheese, cherries, chicken, cranberries, cucumbers

D - dates

E - eggs

F - fennel, figs, filberts, fruit (take care to clean teeth after eating dried fruit and grapefruit)

G - goat's milk, grapes, green beans, green leafy vegetables

H - herring

L - leeks, lentils, lettuce, liver

M - melon, milk, molasses (blackstrap, but be sure to clean teeth after eating)

O - octopus, okra, olives, oranges

P - papaya, parsley, peppers (green and red), pimiento, pistachio nuts, plantains, potatoes, poultry, pumpkin seeds

R - radishes, raspberries

S - sardines, shrimp, spinach, squash, sunflower seeds,
     sweet potato
T - tangerines, tuna, turnips
W - water chestnuts, watermelon
Y - yellow vegetables

Tooth-Cleansing Foods: Especially valuable for between-meal snacking are fruits and vegetables which actually clean the teeth: apples, carrots, celery, and raw zucchini.

Seven

FOOT FACTS

The condition of your feet can encourage or combat wrinkles. It all depends on how they feel and function and the care you give them. When your feet hurt, you seem to hurt all over. The pain shows in your face with tension lines, pinched lips, and pinched eyebrows—all conducive to wrinkles.

One-fourth of all your bones are in your feet—26 to be exact. There are 107 ligaments and 19 muscles. Eons ago when everyone went barefoot and walked on uneven ground, the feet were well exercised. Today they rarely are. And when they are in motion, generally they are hitting hard floors or cement sidewalks and all too often in ill-fitting shoes. If you find a shoe last that really fits you, be loyal. Cherish that manufacturer as you would a dearest friend. He will add joy to your days, health to your life, and help to keep your face free of wrinkles.

Many of us have malformed feet simply because our mothers didn't understand much about them. With the greatest loving kindness, they cramped our feet with too tight sheets, too tight socks, too tight shoes; they carried us around in backpacks that put undue pressure on our feet, and they encouraged us to walk too soon.

According to a doctor in New York City, one of the nation's leaders in the new-age science of kinesiology, too early walking not only often causes malformation of the feet, but produces other physical and psychological problems. If a person did not do enough crawling as an infant, he can mix up left and right, mix up words, be physically awkward, and have other problems too.

Foot exercises: If your shoes are well-fitted, walking is the very best exercise for your feet. The California Longevity Research Institute has documented significant improvements in many ailments by treating patients with a carefully controlled diet and a program of daily walking.

One of the most "fun" exercises for the feet involves picking up your underwear, hose, or any clothes with your toes, without bending your body; but bending your knees, to carry the object to your hand. All of it should be done without bending.

If you don't like dropping your clothing on the floor, you might try the same foot exercise with a batch of sponges. Cut two or three ordinary kitchen sponges into strips or cubes about two inches by two inches. Drop the sponges on the floor, and see if you can pick them up with your toes. Grasping the sponges is fun, and it is excellent exercise.

Foot Care: Wash your feet at least once a day. Dry them carefully, and at least once a week check between your toes to be sure there are no blisters or broken skin. If the skin is broken, you can dust your feet with cornstarch or baby powder.

The skin of your feet, just as other parts of your body, is fed by the blood that is pumped from your heart. And because your feet are so far from your heart, make sure that they are warm, and the dead cells—calluses and corns—are pumiced away. Slathering them with hand lotion is a special treat, and a weekly pedicure will keep them healthy and you much happier.

The pedicure should follow all the steps you usually take for a manicure. The same tools can be used, and you should make sure that you cut your toenails as carefully as you trim and file your fingernails.

Smooth, flexible toes, and a firm strong arch held in comfortable shoes . . . walking along in the fresh air bringing blood to every part of your body is a good way to say, "wrinkles away!"

Part Three

YOUR FACE

Eight

ANTI-WRINKLE FACIAL EXERCISES

In this chapter we present a variety of exercises designed to combat specific problems. You may need to do only a few. You may want to do many. Don't try to start too many exercises the first week. Take it easy. Otherwise your face will get tired and you'll become discouraged. Choose the exercise or exercises that are applicable to the problem that concerns you most.

But remember that some muscles take longer to bring into action. Thus it will take longer for some wrinkles to disappear, while some will go quickly. A small wrinkle is sometimes less responsive than a big one.

Those unattractive vertical lines that appear on the bridge of the nose and between the eyebrows of many women and men is, happily, an easy area for most people to smooth out. That's why it's the first exercise in this chapter.

Do these exercises with a clean, dry face. There are also certain other rules to keep in mind.

1. You must feel relaxed and optimistic and *enjoy* doing the exercises.
2. In those exercises that call for you to use your hands (usually the heels of the palms) or your fingers on your face, be sure that you do not slide or slip hands or fingers over the skin. When the hands or fingers are to be moved from the starting point during an exercise, pick them up and move them.

53

3. Keep in mind that the objective is to *move* the muscle. You can do it in some cases by the muscle itself, directed by the mind. In some cases, you'll use the fingers to move the muscle.
4. Don't continue doing any exercise when your arms become tired. And they will. After all, you will be using your arm in a new way and unless you're a tennis player or golfer, you'll get tired holding your hands to your face.

The exercises that you do should take only a few minutes. In the beginning, you may choose to do them only once a day, but three times a day for the first ten days is better. As you see the benefits, you may want to keep up the three times a day routine for several months —or indefinitely. After all, you'll be creating beauty, and that is a worthy investment of time.

The "smoothings" that follow in the next chapter also are to be done on a daily basis, but only for a limited period. After that you do them whenever you choose. They are a unique facet of this anti-wrinkle program, a facet that is pleasurable and immensely beneficial.

The best time to do these facial exercises is in the morning, after you have washed and dry-patted or air-dried your face and throat. If you decide on the three times a day routine, then the evening is another good time, and you can work in some before dinner. As you *think* about the exercises, you'll find you can do one or two at odd moments during the day and in many places—usually when you're waiting for something or someone.

How old should you be to do these exercises? Any age. You're never too young, nor too old. Teen years is not too young, and we have friends in their eighties who've found wonderful benefit from them.

VERTICAL WRINKLES BETWEEN BROWS

The benefit of this exercise is the elimination of vertical lines between the brows, which have not only an aging effect but an implication of an angry or worried personality.

54

1. Place the index and middle fingers of both hands side by side between the eyebrows, fingers pointing up.
2. Press firmly and massage up and down for a few moments.
3. Now massage horizontally, moving the fingers a little space at a time, about ½ inch from the center out to each brow and back to the center.
4. Massage diagonally up toward the left temple and down toward the right jaw.
5. Massage diagonally toward the right temple and toward the left jaw.
6. Return to center and massage the center area in a circular motion.

CHEEK HOLLOWS

This exercise strengthens large circular muscles around the eyes to prevent or combat sagging. It also strengthens and develops cheek muscles to fill out hollows.

1. Lift corners of lips upward toward the eyes—an exaggerated smile. This contracts, or bunches up, the muscles on the upper part of the cheekbone, directly below the corners of the eyes.
2. Put heels of hands at center of cheeks, using right hand on right cheek, left hand on left cheek.
3. Push heels of hands firmly upward, moving in short movements over contracted muscles toward the temples. (Don't slide your hands.)
4. Relax.
5. Repeat 10 times the first time.
6. After one week, increase to 20 times.

CHEEK MUSCLES

This exercise firms the muscles and rounds the cheeks.

1. Lie on your back on a bed, floor, or slant board.

2. Lift corners of lips upward toward the eyes—an exaggerated smile. This contracts, or bunches up, the muscles on the upper part of the cheekbone directly below the corners of the eyes.
3. Drop chin to lowest point, working against the upward lift of the mouth. This furthers the tension on the cheek-supporting muscles.
4. Keeping the cheek muscles contracted, alternately open and close jaws.
5. While jaws are opening and closing, press cheeks upward with palms of hands from center of cheek to the corner of the eyes and all the way to the hairline above the temples.
6. Relax.
7. Repeat 10 times.

FOR PLUMPER CHEEKS

1. Open mouth into large, tight vertical oval.
2. While holding oval, seek to stretch facial muscles out, up, down into sunflower shape.
3. Hold for count of 5.
4. Relax.
5. Repeat 5 times, morning and evening.

CHEEK CONTOUR

This exercise is good for too thin *or* too fat cheeks. It fills out thin cheeks and firms fleshy ones.

1. Close lips tightly.
2. Fill out and puff cheeks with air.
3. Roll tongue around in each cheek for count of 5 on each side.
4. Relax and exhale.
5. Repeat 5 times.

EYE EXERCISE

This four-part exercise relaxes tension, strengthens eye muscles, and combats wrinkles. It is believed to have originated in ancient China.

1. Press thumbs sideways directly under *eyebrows*, under the bony structure.
2. Push firmly toward the bone.
3. Squeeze eyes shut.
4. Hold for *slow* count of 5.
5. Open eyes slowly.
6. Push up muscles around the eyes.
7. Hold for count of 5.
8. Repeat steps 1 through 7, 4 times.
9. Press thumbs hard against *temples*.
10. Hold for count of 5; relax.
11. Repeat steps 9 and 10, 4 times.
12. Holding thumbs sideways, directly under *center of the eye* sockets, push in firmly.
13. Relax pressure.
14. Repeat steps 12 and 13, 4 times.
15. Press thumbs against *nose* at inner corner of eyes.
16. Push in hard with thumbs held sideways.
17. Relax.
18. Repeat steps 15 through 17, 4 times.
19. Press thumbs hard directly *above center of eyebrow*.
20. Hold press for slow count of 15.
21. Place palms of hands firmly against eyes.
22. Remove quickly.
23. Repeat steps 19 through 22, 4 times.

EYEBROW LIFT

This exercise will combat sagging brows, improve the contour of the lips, and of course improve muscle strength.

1. Open lips slightly.
2. Smile up.

3. Move lips left as far as you can, while lifting left lip corner up toward eyebrow. Note pull on jaw and throat. As you learn to do this properly, you'll see the muscles under the eye socket move with your action.
4. Draw lips back to center. Relax.
5. Repeat exercise to right.
6. Repeat exercise 4 times in both directions.

FACE/NECK EXERCISE

Benefits of this exercise are reduced neck, mouth, and cheek wrinkles, and improved circulation.

1. Open mouth in widest possible oval.
2. Stick tongue out as far as you can.
3. Relax.
4. Repeat steps 1 through 4, 5 times.

NECK EXERCISE

Benefits of this ''chicken peck'' exercise are a firmer and smoother chin, jaw, and throat.

1. Cream neck and throat.
2. Sit, lie, or stand and raise chin.
3. Stretch chin up, *high!*
4. Stretch chin forward, *hard!*
5. Pull head back as far as possible.
6. Repeat forward/back movements as often as desired.

NECK/EYE EXERCISE

Benefits of this exercise are improved circulation, reduced wrinkles, and lessened eye fatigue.

1. Turn head to one side.
2. Look up as high as you can.
3. Look down as far as you can.
4. Relax.
5. Repeat 5 times to the right, 5 to the left.

NECK/SHOULDER/CHIN MASSAGE

This exercise increases circulation, combats double chin, and counter-acts neck wrinkles.

1. Stretch chin up in the air.
2. With the backs of both hands, slap up along the side of the neck, from collarbone to earlobes.
3. Relax.
4. Stretch chin forward and, reaching back with palms of both hands, rub shoulders in a circular motion from lowest point you can reach up to nape of neck.
5. Relax.
6. Repeat as often as desired.

THROAT/SHOULDER/CHIN

This exercise combats double chin and helps fill out hollows above the collarbone.

1. Press palm of one hand flat against forehead.
2. Throw head back as far as you can.
3. Slowly bring head forward until chin touches chest, while resisting with the weight of your hand.
4. Repeat 5 times.

Variation: While head is thrown back, open mouth wide and *chew* vigorously 20 to 30 times.

NOSE-TO-CHIN WRINKLES

This exercise combats nose-to-chin wrinkles, fights double chin, and aids cheek color and tone.

1. Clench lips tight.
2. Blow out cheeks as though trying to force air through the cheeks.
3. While keeping cheeks blown out, pull chin down to force pressure on any present or potential double chin.
4. Hold for count of 5.
5. Relax.
6. Repeat 3 times.

THROAT AND NOSE-TO-MOUTH LINES

1. Grasp center of chin between thumb and index finger.
2. Resisting the effort, pull chin down as far as possible.
3. Continuing resistance, bring chin up as far as it will go, slowly.
4. Relax.
5. Repeat 5 times.

SMOOTHER JAW LINE

Benefits of this exercise are a firmer jaw line and improved circulation.

1. Wring out a light terry hand towel soaked in warm water.
2. Twist towel into a spiral.
3. Slide the towel gently and slowly back and forth along and under the jaw from ear to ear.
4. Keep the towel moist.
5. Repeat as often as desired.

CHIN MUSCLES

Muscles of the chin are involuntary and can be developed only by deep massage that exercises them. This exercise will produce a rounder, firmer chin.

1. Put the heels of the hands together below the center of the chin.
2. Press heels *vigorously* against the jawline upward to earlobes in a firm stroking motion.
3. Relax.
4. Repeat 10 times, relaxing briefly between each upward push.

MOUTH

A wide muscular band encircles the mouth. Unless exercised, this muscle weakens and atrophies with age, causing the mouth to sag and droop at the corners. The following exercises will improve circulation, strengthen muscle tissue, and diminish wrinkles.

MOUTH EXERCISE #1

This exercise combats sag, firms and lifts the mouth.

1. Insert both little fingers into the corners of the mouth.
2. Pull mouth forward with fingers as far as you can, until you feel a weak stretching of the mouth muscle.
3. Hold for *slow* count of 5.
4. Relax.
5. Repeat 10 times.

MOUTH EXERCISE #2

1. Make mouth into large tight O.
2. Tense hard.
3. Hold for slow count of 10.
4. Relax.
5. Repeat 5 times.
6. Do this exercise each morning.

MOUTH EXERCISE #3

This exercise combats vertical lines above the mouth.

1. Make a large O with the lips.
2. Hold cheek and upper lip areas taut.
3. Widen the O as much as you can.
4. Upon reaching the biggest O, hold for a *slow* count of 5.
5. Relax.
6. Repeat 5 times.

MOUTH EXERCISE #4

1. Place fingertips of both hands on upper lip to hold it firm.
2. Make wide O, push *outwards* against your resisting fingertips.
3. Relax.
4. Repeat 5 times.

LIP CONTOUR

Benefits of this exercise are a lift to the lip corners, improved tissue structure, and improved lip texture. If your lips are prone to cracking and peeling, cream them well before attempting this exercise.

1. Open mouth as wide as possible.
2. Insert your little fingers inside corners of the mouth.
3. Stretch mouth as wide as possible with your fingers.
4. Slowly close mouth, resisting with fingers but pulling the fingers together, until fingers meet in the center of the mouth.

TEMPLES

With age, the muscles of the temples are inclined to sink. This exercise combats crow's-feet and fills out temple hollows.

1. Put heels of hands on center of cheekbones.
2. Firmly press in and up, moving the hands in tiny upward lifts to the corners of the eyes and continuing to the hairline, above the temples.
3. Repeat 10 times.

BACK-OF-EAR WRINKLES

Don't neglect the wrinkles that form behind the ears. The skin here, as elsewhere, loosens with age, and short vertical wrinkles form, often extending down to the shoulders.

1. Close teeth, putting tension into jaw/neck areas.
2. Place the index and middle fingers of hands on the bone directly behind the lower part of the ear.
3. Holding fingers firmly in place, push muscle up.
4. Relax.
5. Repeat 10 times, keeping teeth clenched.
6. Repeat, pushing muscle toward the center of the back of the head. Do this 10 times.

WHOLE FACE EXERCISE#1

While most facial exercises work only on one set of muscles at a time, a few strengthen all, including those around the eyes. This two-part exercise will rush new blood to the face to help sweep away old cells and build new ones. It will strengthen muscles of the entire face.

1. Turn eyes in toward bridge of nose. You may be shocked to find you can't do this in the beginning, or that one eye will turn in and the other won't. In time, both will and your eyesight as well as muscle strength will be benefited.
2. Close lips together firmly and pull mouth wide.
3. When you have reached your widest stretch, pull mouth corners *down*.
4. Pull eyebrows down with eyebrow muscles.
5. Tense chin.
6. Hold tension long enough to cause pressure on the weaker tissue cells, to the *slow* count of 5.
7. Release tension.
8. Repeat 2 times.
9. Relax.
10. Close lips firmly and pull wide.
11. When you have reached your widest stretch, lift lip corners *up*.
12. Raise eyebrows as high as possible, opening eyes as wide as possible.
13. Tense chin.
14. Hold lip, eyebrow, eye tension for the *slow* count of 5.
15. Relax.
16. Repeat 2 times.
17. Relax.

WHOLE FACE EXERCISE#2

This exercise specifically attacks wrinkles of the forehead, nose-to-chin lines, double chin, and crow's-feet.

1. Raise eyebrows as high as possible.
2. Open eyes as wide as possible.

3. Lift forehead as high as possible.
4. Draw mouth together tightly into a pursed position.
5. Lower chin to force pressure against any present or potential double chin.
6. Hold for *slow* count of 5.
7. Relax.
8. Repeat 3 times.

WHOLE FACE EXERCISE #3

This exercise benefits facial contour and neck too. The results do not show as quickly as in some of the other exercises but it is an extremely beneficial one. The muscles involved are not accustomed to exercise so that you must mentally *will* the muscles into action.

1. Place the heels of the palms at the temple on each side of the face.
2. Bring the teeth together hard, tightening the muscles of throat, cheek, and jaw.
3. With the heels of the palms, massage in an upward, backward, circulatory motion. Do not allow the hands to slip over the face.
4. Repeat steps 1 through 3, 10 times.
5. After three days, increase to 20 times.
6. If possible do this exercise three times a day.

After your ten-day beauty program, you may increase or decrease the number of times you do this exercise, according to your results and needs.

Your goal is a face that is fresh, smooth, and alive. And it's achievable.

Nine

SMOOTHING WRINKLES AWAY

Now that you know all about wrinkles, how to recognize them, how to combat them with exercises, you are ready to learn how to smooth them away. And for those of you who don't have wrinkles, the method includes prevention as well.

The skin is continually changing and renewing itself and is a constant reflection of the inner being. Prevention and elimination of wrinkles depend upon diet, of course, and exercise, but most important, on keeping the skin moist and soft, and on keeping moisture between the layers of the skin too.

The eye area requires special attention. Since there are fewer layers of skin around the eyes than on any other part of the body, the eye area is particularly susceptible to dryness and therefore to wrinkles. The neck is also very vulnerable to drying skin and wrinkles. Most people never have wrinkles on their nose—the most oily section of the face.

To put the smoothing process to work, you need a private place to work where you have access to a mirror and boiling water. You need:

A light, good oil (can be cold-pressed seed or vegetable oil), or a good, light rejuvenating cream (see Appendix for resource list and recipes).

Some spoons—teaspoon, demitasse spoon, soup spoon, and even a ladle, if you wish—plus a fork and a butter knife.

A mug or two to hold boiling water in which you will heat the spoons.

A small plate.

Boiling water and cold water.

Optional: a tray to hold your equipment; a wooden tray is best because it acts as a heat insulator.

Set up your equipment as if you were getting ready for a light lunch. Place the salad plate in front of you and the spoons to the right and left. If you are right-handed, put the drinking glass at the upper right and the coffee mug at the far right. If you're left-handed, you will find it more comfortable to put drinking glass and mug to the left.

Now you are ready to start. You are going to banish wrinkles by ''ironing'' them away! You will use the back of the bowls of the spoons as your iron, choosing different sized spoons for differently placed wrinkles. The heat and the pressure of ironing will encourage the cream to penetrate the pore to go below the surface layer of skin; there it will stimulate the moisture and circulation, and help ''plump out'' the upper layers.

Even the first ironing can be astonishingly dramatic. Many of you will find your skin will glow, and you may be surprised by the fresh look. Years, and that tired tense look often associated with wrinkles, seem to disappear.

To begin, fill one mug with very hot water. The temperature of most hot water from the tap is just about right. Then fill the other mug with cool water. Put a spoon in the mug of hot water.

Place one teaspoon of cream on the salad plate (use a spatula to remove it from the jar), or if you are using a tubed product, squeeze about an inch of cream from the tube onto your plate.

Starting with your eye area: dot cream directly below each eyebrow, then below the eye, then on the forehead, the cheeks, the chin, the area beneath the nose and around the mouth. Spread the cream over the area adjacent to the cream dots. Try not to stretch the skin, but, instead, press the cream into the skin with the balls of the fingertips. Use the third and fourth fingers. The index fingers sometimes can be too strong for the eye area. Make sure that you cream the ears (including the earlobes), under the chin, and down the neck. Be sure to cream the *back* of the neck as well as the sides and front.

Now what you are going to do is *press* the cream into your skin, using water-heated spoons as your ''presser.'' The heat will maximize the benefit of the cream; the smooth bowl of the spoon will help, as you persist, in diminishing the little wrinkles, performing a smoothing service just as an electric iron smooths the wrinkles from a shirt.

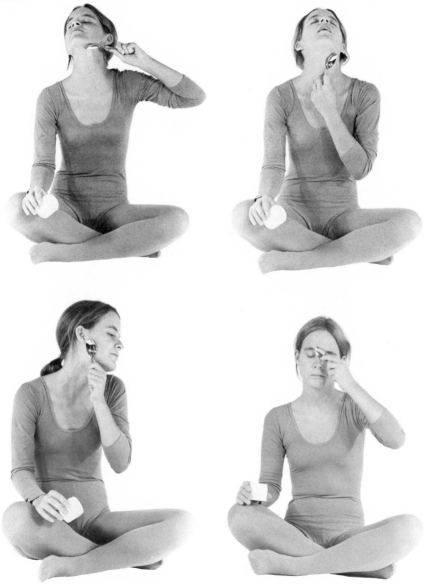

By this time, the spoon that is in the hot water should be well heated. In fact, it may be too hot. If you find the handle is overly hot to your hand, pick it up with a towel and dip it into the cool water mug. Usually one dip will cool it down adequately. Until you learn to gauge the temperature accurately, test the spoon on the back of your hand or on the inside of the elbow, just as you would test a baby's bottle. Your skin should be treated with the same loving, tender care that you'd give a baby!

You are now ready to start a program of and for beauty. The idea behind this program is that *while* you are working toward beauty, you don't have to be ugly. Each day there is some improvement. Mao Tse-tung said, ''The long march starts with the first step,'' and so it does. But how well and rapidly this method works will depend completely on how consistent you are in following the program. Still, the smoothing technique does start to work immediately. Long-term benefits may be possible only after a period of effort, but your mirror will show visible results after only one smoothing. So there is constant support, reassurance, results, and benefits.

As you use the techniques in this section, keep in mind some very basic rules about any exercise program or new beauty technique. Start easy. Work up. A little at first is much better than overdoing. Your body must become attuned to a new technique and your skin should have a chance to react favorably, or unfavorably, to any cream that you might use. Remember that you will be forcing the cream deep into your pores and so into the upper layers of your skin. Watch for an adverse reaction, even from a cream that you have successfully used for years. The idea of the smoothing is to give you a smooth lustrous complexion. Keep trying different creams until you find the one that works best for you.

The authors have used a variety of creams as the lubricant for the smoothing and exercises. A group of volunteers who tried the technique reported that everything from cold cream to olive oil was used successfully as a lubricant. Any vegetable oil that feels agreeable to you will work well. Safflower oil or safflower mayonnaise makes a lovely lubricant. (You'll find recipes in the Appendix.) Safflower mayonnaise is inexpensive, easily cleaned away, easy to store in a refrigerator, and readily available: you can easily make it or use a store-bought product.

Here is a list of do's and don'ts that should be observed:

1. As you exercise and "iron," concentrate on the effects you want.
2. Breath! Sometimes when people are concentrating, they forget to breathe. The idea is to get oxygen into your bloodstream, to help get cleansing and life-giving blood to the freshly exercised and ironed muscles and skin. Adequate oxygen intake is most important.
3. Always apply cream to your hands and wrists as well as to the back of the neck and the area of your neck just under the ears. Don't waste cream, but use enough to ensure a slick surface.
4. Exercise before a well-lighted mirror. Concentrate on what you are doing and notice every push, fold, and motion of the flesh and skin of your face, neck, body, and limbs.
5. You can expect immediate results from the exercises or the smoothing, but keep at it conscientiously for really dramatic results. You'll be surprised how soon you will see dramatic results—benefits that will last for a long time and will not reverse themselves easily.
6. Press the cream that you use into any crease; pat extra cream into the very delicate tissue around the eyes and the neck.
7. Use both hands at the same time. It saves time. You can smooth with two spoons easily, and twice as fast as you can with one.
8. Although your skin varies in texture on different parts of your face and body, remember that it is all connected and very fragile. Treat your skin with tender loving care. It's your most visible part.

69

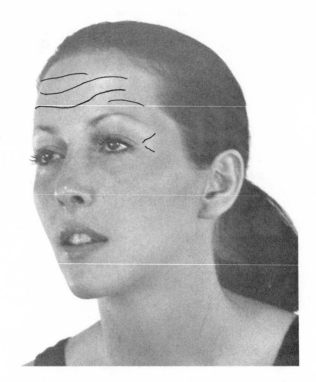

Horizontal Lines on the Forehead

DESCRIPTION

Some wrinkles develop because of use, not because of lack of exercise. Horizontal lines, sometimes called ''worry lines,'' should rightly be called ''expression'' lines. The lines are formed by your raising the eyebrows when talking, gesturing, or thinking.

These lines can be seen on very young faces, sometimes even on teenagers.

PLAN

Look in the mirror and study the lines on your forehead. Notice how they are formed by expression. The goal: to plump out the lines and to smooth away the furrows.

ERASINGS

Lubrication. Cream the entire forehead carefully. Spread the cream from temple to temple, from the brows moving upward to the hairline. *Firming.* Place both hands on the top of the head, with the edges of the hands as close as possible to the hairline. Clench the eyes shut, pulling the muscle of the eye taut. With the forehead muscles, pull down toward the eyebrows and out, toward the temples. Hold for a slow count of three. (You will feel the tension right down to your shoulders.) Open the eyes, and relax the muscles.
Smoothing. With a large soup spoon or a ladle, press and smooth the entire forehead, working downward and outward, and then upward and outward. Because there is a strong hard bone beneath the forehead, press firmly.

FREQUENCY

If you have a tendancy to horizontal wrinkles on your forehead, you will have to iron firmly as often as possible.

Your skull forms a large smooth bone under the skin of the forehead, and that bone will form a good basis for the smoothing. Smooth with the spoon back for at least a minute after creaming; and if possible, smooth for three minutes at each smoothing.

If you have a tendency to get bumps or blackheads on your forehead, remember, these are from improper or faulty outlets to the oil glands, not from the creaming. Wash and brush your forehead often to keep it bump-free; cream and iron it to keep it wrinkle-free.

CAMOUFLAGE

Perhaps the best camouflage is a hair style that covers the forehead. However, you'll find that the forehead lines are less noticeable if you draw the attention *away* from the forehead by putting a focus elsewhere: by dramatizing your eyes, or developing a wonderful smile, or even by wearing a touch of color at the throat, such as a bright scarf. Light-catching earrings also will distract the gaze from a heavily creased forehead.

71

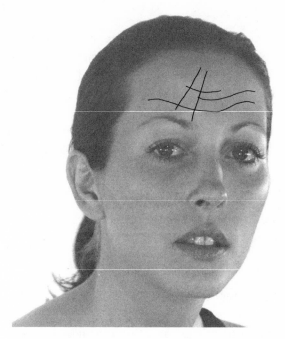

Vertical Lines on the Forehead

DESCRIPTION

The forehead usually hosts horizontal lines that go from temple to temple, but occasionally there are vertical lines that seem to run on an angle from the eyebrows to the hairline. The exercises and smoothings to get rid of these lines are similar to those used to soften frown lines and other vertical lines that might appear on the forehead.

PLAN

The idea is to strengthen the muscle that covers the forehead, the *frontalis* muscle. The technique will include covering and strengthening the muscle and then forcing moisture in the area by smoothing the entire forehead.

ERASINGS

Lubrication. Cover all of the forehead from eyebrows to hairline, from temple to temple. If you are bothered with crow's-feet, apply cream to the entire eye area.

Firming. Place the four fingers of each hand (excluding the thumb) together so that the tips meet. Hold the fingers of each hand on the forehead directly above the eyebrows. Press firmly so that with your fingers you can control the skin on the forehead. Push the skin together and notice how the skin falls into wrinkles and folds. Then, pull the skin sharply apart, so that you are pulling toward each temple. Push the skin together again. Now, using only muscles of the forehead, try to push your fingers away from each other toward the temples, working against the resistance of the fingers.

Smoothing. Heat a large soup spoon to slightly warmer than body temperature. Using the back of the bowl of the spoon as a smoother, follow the vertical lines on the forehead. You can press rather hard since there is a firm hard bone over the forehead.

FREQUENCY

Forehead lines are difficult to remove. You will probably have to iron the lines at least two times a day for at least two weeks before there is a real change in appearance. You must also avoid scowling absentmindedly, or keeping the fingers on the forehead, or resting your hand against your head when you are reading or working.

CAMOUFLAGE

Of course bangs will camouflage all lines on the forehead, but if you look best with your hair away from your forehead, it would be good to wear it that way. Avoid hair ornaments, incandescent eye shadows, or extreme eye makeup that brings attention to this area of the face. Be sure that your hairline is clean and neat and that wisps of hair do not hang over your forehead and cause a disheveled appearance.

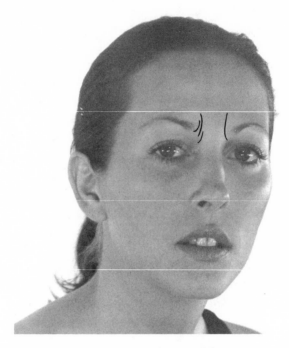

Vertical Lines Between Eyebrows: Scowl

DESCRIPTION

Scowl lines are expression lines; you cannot blame age, face shape, or even dry skin. These lines are formed by your pulling the brows together. Young people, even teenagers, often have small scowl lines. They can give the face a very unfriendly expression.

PLAN

Because you only form the scowl lines, you can rid yourself of them quite easily and quickly. The first step is to learn to control the muscles that form the scowl. When you can control those muscles, the rest will be easy. Using the smoothing technique, you can force moisture into the outer skin and mitigate the vertical lines.

ERASINGS

Lubrication: Cream the scowl area, extending the cream over the forehead and to the ends of the brows.

Firming: Standing before the mirror, practice bringing your brows together and then apart. The trick is to separate the brows and flatten the scowl marks without raising the eyebrows. Move the brow muscles as slowly as possible. Counting to yourself, move the brows until you feel tired.

Smoothing: Using a very large soup spoon or a flat, round-bowled spoon, press the back of the spoon against each scowl line as you move overriding skin. Use the iron in an outward motion, working toward each temple. You can use a spoon in each hand and work on both scowl lines at the same time.

FREQUENCY

Elimination of scowl lines requires continual ironing from without, and *conscious* change in expression control. It is easy to say don't scowl, but hard to break the habit. However, you *can* remember to use sunglasses and to avoid close work without proper lighting, and it is possible to form the habit of *not* expressing displeasure with a hard, firm glance—a scowl.

CAMOUFLAGE

Use sunglasses or tinted glasses with a wide nosepiece.

If it is flattering, wear a hair style that exposes the top of the ear. Otherwise, draw attention to the outer edges of the face with a decorative comb or pin.

Wear a hat with a generous brim. Be sure that the brim sits far away from the brows and that the angle of the hat tilts upward.

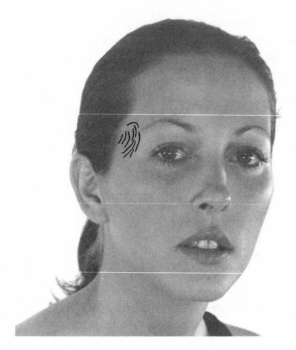

Sides of the Temple

DESCRIPTION

When the skin on the sides of the face dries and the under-muscles slacken, the problem is a difficult one. The skin at the temple between the eye and the hairline is just such a difficult spot. In later years the skin in this area is often very dry, and because it is so near the delicate eye and the hairline, it is sometimes ignored in cleansing and in moisturizing. The slight sag in the dry skin makes any small lines around the eyes look even worse. This area is usually one of the first tightened in surgical face-lifting.

PLAN

The first job is to identify the muscles under the skin. The muscle belt around the eye, called the *orbicularis oculi,* is the major muscle group. This circular muscle belt can be toned up by pulling and tugging, tightening the entire eye area.

ERASINGS

Lubrication. Cream the entire area around the eye. Spread the cream from the outer edge of the eye to the hairline. Be sure that the forehead and the temple area above the eye are also creamed.

Firming. Strengthening and firming the eye muscles is difficult. And the misuse of the scalp muscles, the *temporal fascia* that control the entire over-ear area, makes it even more difficult. Close your eyes, and tighten both eyes as much as possible. Pull the lids together. Place your fingers on the temple area and note how you can feel the muscles pulling toward the eye. Now, with the eye muscles still tightened, pull back on the scalp muscles. Try to move your ears and the scalp over the ears back and forth. Practice can teach you control of the eye area.

Tighten, pucker, pull-back. Repeat this five times, working on both temple areas at once. When you tighten the muscles, try to hold the pulled-together lids for the count of three, then pull back on the scalp muscles as sharply as possible.

Smoothing. Using a small teaspoon or demitasse spoon, work the sagging skin from the eye area toward the hairline. Work upward and outward urging the cream into the flesh and skin as you go. There is a firm bone over much of the forehead, but the temple area is quite delicate and care should be taken so that the pressure of the smoothing does not dilate and press the delicate blood vessels and cause a headache.

FREQUENCY

If the temple area is noticeably wrinkled, repeat the exercise and smoothing techniques at least three times a week for at least four weeks. You should notice improvement after about two weeks, but do not stop. After about four weeks a once-a-week maintenance program will keep your eyes open and sparkling and make an upswept ''off the face'' hairdo possible.

CAMOUFLAGE

A hair style that is soft and delicate on the sides of the face can cover the temple area. Or, a hair style that pulls the hair up to the top of the scalp has the effect of providing an ''instant face-lift.'' However, tightening the temple hair weakens the hair follicles and can eventually cause the loss of hair.

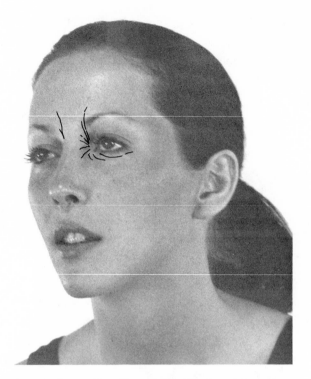

Scowl at the Bridge of the Nose

DESCRIPTION

The lines that appear slightly inside each of the eyebrows, directly over the nose and between the eyes, are unfortunate and make a face seem hard and unpleasant. The lines also might affect the skin at the bridge of the nose on either side of the nose, with a series of tiny lines spreading from the inner corner of the eye to the nose.

PLAN

Strengthening the muscles on either side of the nose can be done by controlling the muscle that controls the eyebrows. But to do this, the muscles must be trained to react against a force or resistance.

ERASINGS

Lubrication. Apply cream very liberally to the entire eye area and to the upper part of the cheeks. Also cream the forehead lightly.

Firming. Place your index fingers at the base of the scowl lines, on either side of the nose. Press firmly. Concentrating on the center of the forehead, move the muscles of only the center of the forehead up and out. Try not to move the fingers; rather use the two firmly held index fingers to control the muscles. You should be able to feel the pull and pressure of the muscles under your index fingers.

Smoothing. The affected area of the inner eye and the top and bridge of the nose is very difficult to reach with any but the smallest demi-tasse spoon. Use a tiny spoon—the flatter the bowl, the better—and with the back of the spoon, smooth the creases on either side of the bridge of the nose. Work from the top of the nose in, but be careful not to get any cream into the eye. Then work from the inner eye to the top of the nose and up into the forehead. Smooth each side at least five times.

FREQUENCY

Repeat the exercise at least five times each exercise session and repeat the exercise sessions at least once daily for a week. The smoothing should follow each of the exercise sessions.

A maintenance program of about twice a week and then after you've hit a plateau, once a week can be used to keep once-erased wrinkles away forever.

CAMOUFLAGE

Do not call attention to the upper nose and bridge of the nose area by fingering that part of the face. Avoid eye shadow that is brought too close to the inner edge of the eye. If you wear glasses, choose a style with a large bridge. Do not wear hats or scarves that call attention to the brow area by ending just above the eyebrows.

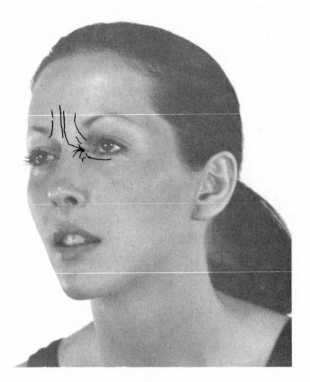

Lines at the Bridge of the Nose

DESCRIPTION

Lines across the bridge of the nose are rare in a face that is younger than 50 years. They are usually due to the bad habit of knitting the brows, or to squinting when doing especially close work. Many wrinkles can be avoided if you get into the habit of having your eyes examined regularly.

PLAN

Smoothing the lines at the bridge of the nose can be done only by controlling the under-muscles across the top of the nose, being sure that the skin is kept soft and pliable. You may want to use a tissue when doing this exercise to be sure creamed skin does not slip when you are exercising against a resistance.

80

ERASINGS

Lubrication. Cream the entire eye area and spread cream down the sides of the nose. Cream forehead as well.

Firming. Hold the top of the nose with the fingers of the right hand (if you are right-handed). With the muscles of the brow, push up and out. Exercise the brow muscles by pushing and holding the muscles.

Smoothing. Use a small demitasse spoon. Hold the skin around the top of the nose and press the bowl of the tiny spoon against the skin, starting at the middle of the nose. Do not use spoon on tip of nose— especially if it is oily. Work up the nose, gliding the back of the bowl and then to the lower forehead. You can press firmly since there is a strong bone under the area. However, be sure that the spoon is small enough for you to get into the area near the eye.

FREQUENCY

It will take a long time to erase or even lessen the lines over the nose. Keep smoothing, for perhaps two or three weeks before you notice any improvement. After that a maintenance schedule of at least four times a week, or every other day, will be necessary. And, of course, it is necessary to avoid the expression that first encouraged the lines— a scowl.

CAMOUFLAGE

A pair of glasses—perhaps pretty sunglasses—with a large bridge, or an ''aviator style'' pair of glasses might do very well to keep anyone from noticing the lines, until they disappear completely.

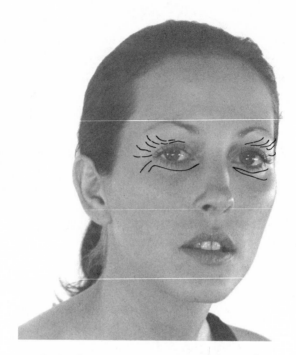

Overhanging Upper Eyelids

DESCRIPTION

An aging face almost always shows droopy eyebrows and a weakening of the skin over the eye. The effect is sometimes called the "lazy eye." Since we see only the skin, we assume that it is the skin that hangs, but actually it is the muscles that need strengthening. Special care must be taken in smoothings because of the sensitivity of the skin in this area.

PLAN

The goal is to open the eye and give the face a brighter, more open look. This can be done by firming up the muscles that attach the upper lid and the brow. Then, we smooth the area, forcing moisture into the sensitive skin surrounding the area.

ERASINGS

Lubrication. Cream the entire eye area carefully. Cream the forehead as well, especially creases. Avoid getting cream into the eye.

Firming. Study the area of the upper eye. Does the skin seem softer and droopier on the outer edge, or on the inner edge, near the nose? Moving the muscles and skin will supply fresh blood to the appropriate area and will firm and brighten the entire eye. Several times a day, open the eyes as wide as possible. Trying not to move the forehead, move the muscles of the upper eyelids, first upward, then downward. It is easier to move the muscles downward since that can be done by *puckering the eyelids together.* Move the eyebrow area up, up, up, then in three movements down and puckering. Repeat ten times.

Smoothing. Place a small heated demitasse or tiny baby spoon firmly against the creamed skin of the upper eyelids. Press the little spoon repeatedly against the eyelid, moving the spoon outward in tiny steps, to press the moisture into the delicate upper eye area. Do not drag the spoon across the eyelid.

FREQUENCY

The eye responds best to frequent but short exercises. Press the smoothings for no more than five minutes each evening for about a week. After that, you should restrict each exercise period to a minute or two, but you may increase the exercise periods to two or more times a day. You can even exercise the eyelids on the street, if you wear sunglasses and keep your eyelids creamed.

CAMOUFLAGE

Take care that the eyebrows are carefully plucked; if the hair on the brows is excessively long or unruly, trim it carefully with a manicure scissors. If your brows are very dark, you might want to consider bleaching. Light brows do not attract attention to the brow area.

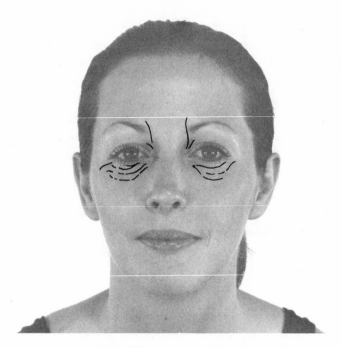

Circles and Bags under Eyes: Lower Lids

DESCRIPTION

Circles and lines under the eyes are due to the lengthening of the muscles of the lower lid. The skin is very sensitive in this area and easily becomes dry. Puffiness can be due to allergy to cosmetics, sinus trouble, or a faulty kidney. It is difficult to encourage circulation of the blood in this area, but as with other wrinkles, good blood circulation is key to their erasure.

PLAN

Strengthening the muscles of the eyelids and smoothing the creases that are in the lower lid can ''open the eye'' and achieve a younger look. The goal can be accomplished with surprising speed.

ERASINGS

Lubrication. Cover the eye area with a complete, but thin, coat of cream. Avoid getting grease or cream into the eye.

84

Firming. Squeeze both eyes shut in a lid-puckering motion. Draw the puckered lids toward the nose. Hold for the count of three. Relax eyelids so that you can pull them to the outer corners of each eye. Relax closed lids, holding eyeball still beneath them. Seek to move closed lids outward, toward the temples. Repeat five times.

Smoothing. With a very small spoon, starting at the inner part of the eye, near the nose, smooth the skin on the lower lid. Work toward the outer corner of the eye. Be sure the area is heavily creamed. Take care not to drag the spoon across the delicate tissue; Slide the spoon, gliding in the cream. At the outer eye corner smooth upward toward the temple.

FREQUENCY

Results will come very quickly if you use the techniques every night for seven consecutive nights. Then reduce to about three or four times a week. Too much manipulation before the muscles start to firm themselves might actually do damage. So remember, daily (or nightly) for one week, then no oftener than three or four times a week.

CAMOUFLAGE

Obviously the best camouflage is dark or colored glasses. Glasses with brown, tan, or light gray tint seem to be attractive on most people. Avoid pink or purple shaded lenses since these make the eyes look bleary.

Bright colored lipstrick—a clean, sharp orange-red—is good on every complexion except the most ruddy. It will draw attention to the mouth and away from the eyes.

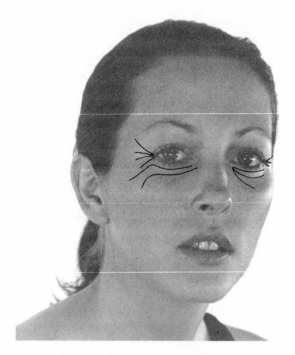

Lines at the Corner of the Eye: Crow's-Feet

DESCRIPTION

Lateral creases that appear on the outer edges of the eyes as early as age 30, and even earlier for smokers, are called ''crow's-feet.'' Clawlike, they deepen with squinting. They are common in men or women who do not wear sunglasses when they work, play, or exercise regularly in bright light outdoors.

PLAN

Because there is a strong, hard bone beneath the ''wrinkled area'' on the outer edge of the eye, the wrinkles can be ironed away more easily than most people would think. It requires diligent ironing for several days, but results will be astonishing.

ERASINGS

Lubrication. Cream the entire eye area. Put emphasis on the outer eye.

Firming. There is very little muscle beneath the outer eye and temple area. It is the area that is most effected by ''crow's-feet.'' This makes firming techniques, with the emphasis on muscle development, almost impossible. The most important part of the erasing proceedure is the penetration of the creams into the very delicate skin.

Stand in front of the mirror, and carefully cream the face, especially the eye area. Pull back on the eye muscle as much as possible, opening the eyes very wide to a startled expression.

Hold each startled expression to the count of three. Then relax, and repeat. Exercise the muscles for firming at least three times before attempting to smooth away the crow's feet with the ironing technique.

Smoothing. Use a small teaspoon or a dessert spoon that has a rather flat bowl. Rub the heated spoon over the wrinkled area with an outward motion, from the edge of the eye to the temple. Work down the cheek from the area over the eye to the skin near the top of the ear. After one ironing for about ten smoothings on each eye area, recream the skin.

FREQUENCY

Iron and smooth the wrinkled area every day, preferably twice daily, until results are seen. Avoid grimacing, squinting, and sunlight. If you have crow's-feet and are under 30 years of age, or if the crow's-feet are very deep, you might well consider having a doctor check your vision.

CAMOUFLAGE

Smiling helps. It is natural to have small creases around the eyes when laughing or smiling. They appear even on a child's face. A happy, contented expression will also help to soften the fine cracks and faults around the eyes.

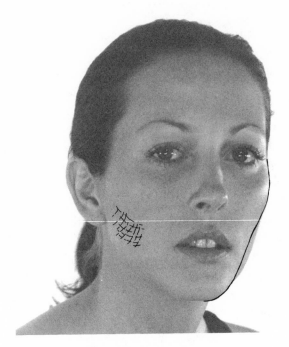

Sides of the Cheek

DESCRIPTION
When the muscles on the side of the face lengthen and weaken, a depression is noticeable in front of the ear, slightly over the jawline. This hollow contributes to making a person look tired and old. The entire face looks soft and sad.

PLAN
Fill the sides of your cheeks with air and puff out gradually. You'll notice that there is a great deal of space on the sides of your mouth between your cheek and your teeth. It is this cheek area that must be firmed. There is a muscle and fat pad that actually forms the cheek— a covering over the sides of your teeth, just where your molars are. It will be necessary to form and tighten the muscles and the skin over the muscles in the pads.

ERASINGS
Lubrication. Cream both sides of your face from mouth to ear. Apply the cream upward past the eye to the temple area.

Firming. This exercise will require you to place your index fingers in your mouth. Place your two index fingers, one on each side of your cheek over your teeth. Place the fingers as far back as possible so that they cover your wisdom teeth or your last set of molars. Using all the strength of your cheek and jaw muscles, try to force your fingers against your teeth as firmly as possible. Squeeze your muscles together so that the fingers are held securely on the side of the teeth. Hold this position to the count of ten; then relax.

Smoothing. Using a large soup spoon, gently caress the area on the side of the face from the jaw upward to the eye area, and then from the mouth over to the side of the face toward the ear. The smoothing will force moisture into the upper layers of the skin and make the skin seem glossy, smooth, and vital. The firming of the underlying muscles will bring a youthful look to your cheeks in about two weeks, if you firm and smooth two or three times a week.

FREQUENCY

Exercise and firm every day for the first two weeks. Then continue a maintenance program of twice a week.

CAMOUFLAGE

Applying a lighter shade of makeup or using a bit of light or white eye shadow in the hollow area of the cheek will visually puff it out until the firmings and smoothings improve the area. Use light colors near your face and avoid calling attention to the area with elaborate earrings or hair styles that end at mid-cheek.

Starting with the forehead, place the *back* of the spoon near your hairline and carefully iron the cream into your face, ironing your wrinkles away. The spoon should be comfortably hot and should be reheated in the hot water as soon as it starts to cool off.

A good rule to remember is always to smooth from the deepest part of a wrinkle to the end of the wrinkle.

It does not matter if you iron across or in the direction of the wrinkle, or in a circular motion. The heat, the smoothing action, the ''iron'' surface, are what count. Experiment with butter knives, forks, and other silver serving utensils as ironers. Often the back of the spoon does the very best job in a small area.

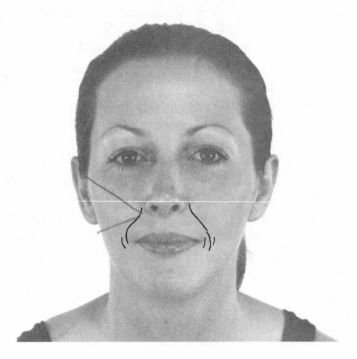

Furrows from Nose to Mouth: Laugh Lines

DESCRIPTION

The largest muscle in the face is the muscle group around the eye. The eye is attached to the mouth with a series of strip muscles. When they lengthen, the cheek droops. A sagging cheek, and the drying of the skin between the nose and mouth, cause the charmingly called, uncharming looking "laugh lines." If the teeth are large or shaped in a convex structure, laugh lines can appear quite early.

PLAN

Exercise the muscles that attach the cheek and side of the face to the lip to firm the cheek and smooth contours. Notice that the corner of the nose is almost directly under the inner eye. Mentally draw an invisible line from the mouth to the *outer eye*, and another from the mouth to the earlobe and sides of the face. This is the area to firm.

ERASINGS

Lubrication. Cream the entire face area and side of face. Spread cream from the upper lip across the cheek to the earlobe. A good covering is needed.

Firming. Place the edges of your teeth together so the front teeth meet. Keeping your mouth as relaxed as possible (do not clinch teeth; just keep them touching), use your facial muscles to pull your cheeks forward. At first it seems an impossible task, but don't be discouraged. The muscles are voluntary and can be moved at will.

Smoothing. Using a teaspoon or dessert spoon, iron the cheek, starting at the corner of the mouth and working outward from the bottom of the nose to the ear, working in gentle, horizontal, side-by-side pressings. Iron only out. Start again at the side of the nose slightly above the initial point and again press *out.* Repeat movement, stepping spoon upward each time until you reach the top of the laugh line. Keep the area well creamed and press the spoon *firmly* against the skin, *urging* the cream into the dried skin. Do not *drag* the spoon back and forth across the crease.

FREQUENCY

Press and iron gently every night for three or four nights. Then use the smoothing techniques every other night for about a month. For maintenance, smooth the area twice weekly. The frequency really depends on the condition of your own skin and underlying muscles. You may need to smooth daily for a few weeks, but you will find the rewards well worth it.

CAMOUFLAGE

Avoid wearing your hair on your cheeks. This tends to call attention to the small area around the mouth. Bright, light-catching earrings and a hairdo that draws attention to the outer edges of the face are good. Light or white collars, soft silk scarves on the shoulders, and pearls worn lower than the collarbone all are good camouflage devices.

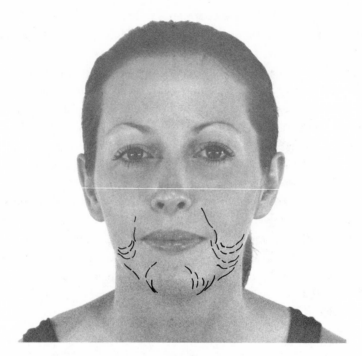

Pouches on the Lower Cheek

DESCRIPTION

Those darling little pouches on the sides of the face look wonderful on squirrels, but not on humans. If you look at the side of your face in the mirror, you will be able to tell if you are a victim of the elongation of the upper cheek muscles—the *zygomatics* muscle—and bear the resulting lower cheek pouch.

PLAN

The idea of firming is based on the strengthening of the muscles that grow longer and allow the pouches to form on the side of the face. The muscle that needs to be strengthened is the *triangularis*.

ERASINGS

Lubrication. Cover the entire lower face with cream. Cream the throat and neck.

Firming. Place the teeth and lips together in a relaxed position. Lift the corners of the mouth toward the temples. Smile purposefully, pulling the outer corners of the mouth up and out. Slowly return the outer corners of the mouth to the natural position. Do this as slowly as possible, controlling the muscles as you release them.

Smoothing. Using a teaspoon or other small spoon, carefully slide it along the skin from the outer corner of the mouth, up the side of the cheek toward the tip of the ear.

FREQUENCY

Exercise the muscles and smooth the skin over the area three or four times a week.

CAMOUFLAGE

Avoid dangling earrings or a busy collar ornament.

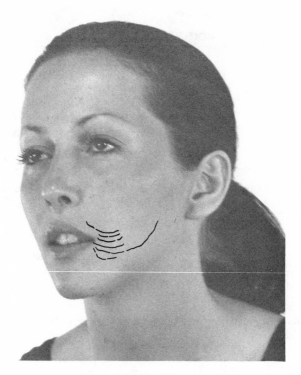

Lower Cheeks and Corners of the Mouth

DESCRIPTION

Often quite early in life a small line will appear next to the corner of the mouth. The fine line, probably no more than a quarter of an inch long, is exactly parallel to the corner edges of the mouth. Together with these lines, and seeming to radiate from them, appear to be a series of soft skin pouches that are almost flabby-looking. If you had a dimple in early life, this dimple may now be turning into a vertical crease. This is a sign of the elongation of the muscles through age and lack of tone.

PLAN

The hope is to strengthen the muscles in the lower cheek. It is easiest and quickest to do this by exercising against a pressure or resistance. You should use the index fingers of both hands to do this. Place the index fingers just inside the inner edge of the corners of the mouth. With the thumb and the index finger, note the flesh and muscle pad that begins just inside the corner of the mouth. It is that pad that must be firmed and toned. We will do this by expanding and contracting the muscles in the mouth and cheek area. The lower cheek will be stressed.

ERASINGS

Lubrication. Cream the entire lower part of the face. Stress the corners of the mouth and the cheek area just beside the corners of the mouth. *Firming.* Place the index fingers on the inner corners of your mouth. Place the first joint of the finger inside the area, and push the smile lines out with your fingers.

Grip the edges of the cheeks with the thumbs and the index fingers. The skin should be firmly held slightly outward from the teeth. Pull the skin forward, as if you would like to force the outer corners of each edge of the mouth to meet.

When you have pulled as much as possible, use only the muscles of the cheek and mouth and try to pull the edges apart. The pull of the muscles should be toward each ear.

Repeat the exercise: first unnaturally bring the corners of the mouth together (the lips will, of course, go up and out), and then, using the muscles of the mouth, try to pull the corners apart.

Smoothing. After exercising the muscles, the skin of the mouth will be warm and very receptive to smoothing. Use only a very small spoon. Work the cream from the outer corners of the mouth toward the ear. Be sure not to forget the lower lip; smooth the skin under the lip from the center of the face outward. Work up and out.

FREQUENCY

This simple and very effective exercise followed by the smoothing technique should be repeated at least three times a week for several weeks, or until the area loses any ''pauchy'' effect and is firm and plump. Then a maintenance program of once a week will be sufficient.

CAMOUFLAGE

It is almost impossible to disguise the soft pouchy area next to the mouth. The best camouflage is often to draw attention to another part of the face, such as the forehead. Avoid very dark sunglasses; this would force anyone who sees you to concentrate on the mouth area since they would not be able to see your eyes.

Another possible disguise would be to use a light foundation or powder just outside the inner corner of the mouth. It would have the visual effect of bringing that area forward, making the skin appear firmer.

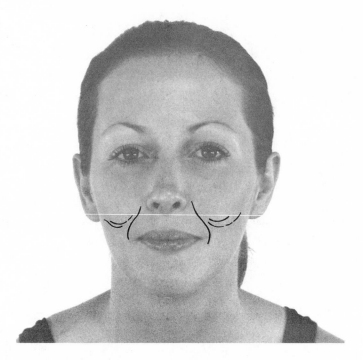

Smiling as an Exercise

DESCRIPTION

There is nothing as youthful and attractive as a sparkling, lovely smile. But when the muscles weaken and the skin dries, small pouches sometimes appear on the sides of the mouth, and these detract from the charm of an inviting smile.

PLAN

This is an easy exercise, and results should be easy to see very quickly. The plan is to exercise and tighten the muscles of the edges of the mouth and the sides of the cheek. All of these muscles are needed when you smile. Good control over the muscles is essential.

ERASINGS

Lubrication. Cream the entire mouth and cheek area. Be sure the cream covers the upper lip, the area between the nose and lip, and the side of the cheek.

Firming. Strengthening and tightening the muscles can be done most easily by pulling the muscles against a resistance. The most practical resistance is your own fingers. Place your index fingers in your mouth, the nails next to the teeth, the finger cushion toward the cheek. Taking care not to injure your gums, slide your fingers along the teeth between the teeth and the inside of the mouth. Then, using both hands at once, after the fingers are placed as far back as they can go, pull the cheeks taut against the index fingers. Try to bring the edges of the mouth as close together as possible, and pull the corners of the mouth together trying to close the mouth.

Smoothing. Use both a large spoon and a teaspoon. With the smaller spoon, smooth the area under the nose by circling the area around the mouth, paying special attention to the corners of the mouth. Then, switching to the larger spoon, carefully press and slide the warm spoon along the cheek from the mouth to the ear. The spoon should glide along the cheek area.

FREQUENCY

Repeat the tightening exercise three or four times before smoothing. Then smooth with spoons three or four times. Repeat the exercise once a day for about a week. Then, for maintenance, exercise and smooth only three times a week.

CAMOUFLAGE

Don't stop smiling. A twinkling eye, a pleasant and snappy look, and a flattering hair style of smooth, shining, clean locks will detract from any soft area around the mouth. Avoid very dark lipstick and be sure that the lipstick is applied with a brush so that the line is clean and straight. You may want to experiment with lip pencils to get a neat clear line, especially in the corners of the mouth. A glossy lipstick, or lip gloss over your favorite lipstick, might brighten your entire mouth area.

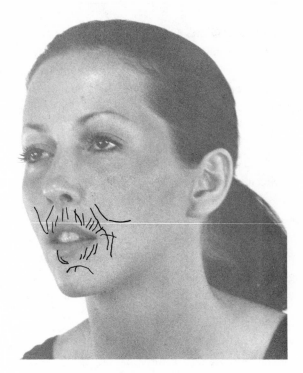

Contour in the Upper Lip

DESCRIPTION

Creases that radiate from the upper lip toward the nose seem to form on some faces but not on others that are equally old or dry. Dr. Michael Marder, a well-known New York dentist, suggests that a thinning of the upper lip as well as missing or poorly fitting teeth might be the cause. These marks show equally on smokers and nonsmokers. A full, soft upper lip is youthful and appealing.

PLAN

You can exercise the muscle of the upper lip, the *obicularis oris*, by tensing it against the upper teeth. It is very easy and effective, and the small wrinkles do respond almost immediately.

ERASINGS

Lubrication. Cream the upper lip, the sides of the mouth, and the cheek area including the base of the nose.

Firming. Open the mouth forming an oval and then pull your lip down so that the actual lip area is curled under the upper teeth and lower teeth.

Pull the sides of the mouth out to force the lip flat against the upper teeth. Using the upper teeth as a resistance, pull back, using the cheek muscles, and hold the lip firmly against the teeth for the count of three.

Relax, and exercise again.

Smoothing. After exercising the upper lip, use a demitasse spoon to smooth the entire area. Pay special attention to the edge of the lip where it meets the skin. Work the wrinkles from the lip out toward the nose, cheek, and jaw.

FREQUENCY

Exercise the upper lip often. If you do notice any small wrinkles after examining the upper lip closely, you should exercise every day for the first week, and then about three times a week for maintenance for the next several weeks. A real improvement should be noticeable after only a week.

CAMOUFLAGE

The use of a lipstick brush or a lip pencil is essential. You will notice that lipstick seems to smear and blob so it is difficult to get a smooth, sharp edge. If you cover the lip with powder before applying lipstick, the color will remain clear and will stay on.

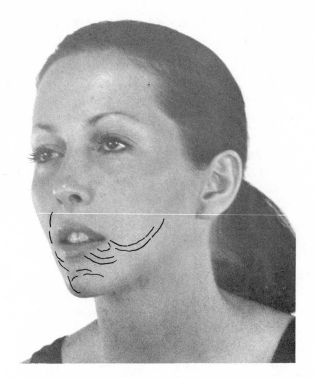

Lines and Sags on Lower Lip, and Unfirm Chin

DESCRIPTION

The *orbicularis oris* is the large circular beltlike muscle that circles the mouth. The muscles of the upper lip and the lower lip usually atrophy at the same time; the flesh pad becomes thinner, and the lips and chin take on a sunken and shrunken look. The wrinkles seem to fold over the chin and the skin looks crepey.

PLAN

To restore the full youthful contour of the lips and chin, you must exercise the underlying muscle. This is done from the inside of the mouth and the outside of the chin. In both exercises, your muscles will be trained to work against a resistance.

ERASINGS

Lubrication. Spread cream over the entire mouth and chin area. Be sure the chin and under-chin area are covered.

Firming. Place the two index fingers inside the mouth in front of the lower teeth. With the index fingers push the lower lip out. Pull the mouth muscles against the fingers so that the fingers form a resistance against the lip muscles. Pull and squeeze the muscles against the fingers three times. Relax, and then repeat the exercise.

Now, place your index fingers on each side of your chin. The fingers should be just under the lower corners of the lips. Push the fingers together so that the flesh of the middle of the chin is pushed together. Then, using the chin muscles only, try to push the fingers apart. Repeat this three times. Relax, and then repeat the exercise again.

Smoothing. You will need a small dessert spoon or a very small soup spoon as a smoother. Working from the middle of the chin outward, smooth the skin on first one then the other side of the mouth and work the cream into the edge of the lower lip. Do not forget the outer corners of the lips.

FREQUENCY

Exercise the lower lip and chin once a day for at least one week. A maintenance program of once-a-week will be needed to keep the chin firm and flexible.

CAMOUFLAGE

Calling attention to the lower lip by biting the lip, fingering the chin, resting your fingers on your chin, or even allowing your lips to fall slack will have the effect of attracting attention to your chin. Avoid dark-colored or messy lipstick; it also will call attention to the lower lip and chin.

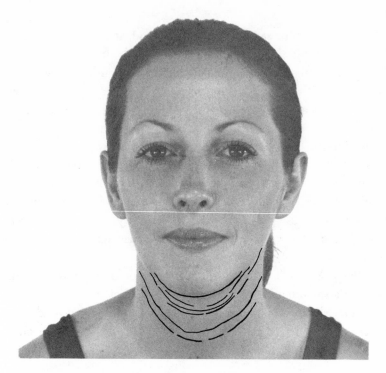

Flabby Muscles Under the Chin: Double Chin

DESCRIPTION

As early as the second decade of life, many people notice that the skin on the bottom of their chin seems loose and saggy. This is especially evident when seen from profile. A tight, clean, and sharp jawline is a mark of health and vigor.

PLAN

Touch the area under the chin firmly and notice that the jawbone defines the outer edge of the face. Soft tissue and muscles seem to be kept in their proper place only by a thin tissue of muscles and skin. It is these muscles that must be firmed, and the skin over the muscles that should be ironed into smooth sleekness.

102

ERASINGS

Lubrication. Cream the entire neck area from ear to ear. Use upward and outward motions, working from the middle of the throat to the ear.

Firming. Place the back of your hand under your chin. Tense your chin muscles, pushing down against your hand. Do not allow your hand to move, but, with tongue held firmly against your teeth and mouth shut, push downward using only the muscles of your chin to try to move the hand. You will be pushing against the resistance of your hand. Do this ten times.

Smoothing. Taking a large, smooth soup spoon for your iron, stroke the skin on the bottom of your chin using a neck-to-chin direction, and middle neck to under-ear direction. Use a firm even motion. Tense your muscles against the spoon as you smooth.

FREQUENCY

While the neck and chin seem to "go first," they also respond well to care and exercise. The smoothing by the iron and the firming of the muscles should bring some results in about ten days. In about two weeks some definite improvement should be evident.

CAMOUFLAGE

Keeping the skin on the neck protected from cold winds, sun, and drying is important. There are few oil glands on the neck, and it is an area of strain. Scarves are great flatterers. Moisturizers by day and emollients by night will work together with exercise and ironing.

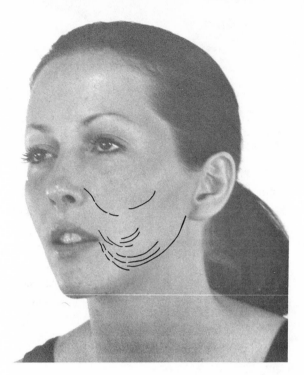

Jowls

DESCRIPTION

The soft saggy pockets that form on the bottom of the jaw are usually called jowls. While they are a sign of good breeding in hunting dogs, they are a no-no for people. They come from the muscles of the cheek elongating and losing strength. The muscles seem to slide to the bottom of the face and drag overlying skin with them, causing the bulge.

PLAN

The idea is to exercise the *triam-gularis* muscle and to control the cheek muscles so that they will support their share of facial weight. The job will be two-part: pulling the muscle and jowl up, and then training the cheek muscle.

ERASINGS

Lubrication. The entire face must be creamed; this is a most active exercise. Spread the cream evenly on the face and carefully on the neck. Be sure that the mouth, cheek, and jaw areas are covered and softly lubricated. Carefully lubricate the neck as well.

Firming. Pretend you have an underbite; bring your lower teeth out and up, trying to grasp your upper lip with your bottom teeth. Try to bring your bottom lip up, holding it firmly against the upper teeth and covering the bottom teeth, which are on top of the upper teeth. This will give you a bulldog look.

Be sure that there is enough cream on the lower jaw area. Now, holding the upper lip firmly but gently between your teeth with the jaw out, concentrate on smiling: bring both lip corners up in a smile position. If this is too difficult, first smile on one side, then the other.

Try tilting the edge or outer corner of the mouth toward the tip of the ear on that side; smile by pulling and pulling the muscles up to the sides of the face, using both outer lip and cheek muscles.

Repeat the exercise ten times on each side of the face. You might find it easier to do one cheek at a time at first, and then both at the same time.

Smoothing. Using the back of a teaspoon or a small soup spoon, smooth the skin on the jowl and lower jaw area. The area that should be smoothed is very large, from the chin to the upper ear, and down below the jaw on the neck. All of the skin must be moisturized. Add more cream if it seems necessary. Carefully, with round circular motions urge the cream into the upper layers of the skin. Use a rotary motion and try to avoid dragging the skin. If the skin is very loose, hold the section that you are smoothing with your fingers. Use your left hand to hold your skin if you use the spoon in your right hand.

FREQUENCY

This exercise and smoothing will take a long time; repeat ten times each side per session. The first week, you should exercise and smooth directly after the exercising at least once a day for three to five minutes. After that about three times a week will be sufficient.

CAMOUFLAGE

High, tight turtleneck sweaters, severe prints, necklaces that call attention to the jaw area, and long dangling earrings should be avoided. A light-colored, soft, open collar or a very colorful scarf that draws the eye to the shoulders, or other camouflages are good. Never tie anything under the chin, since even a scarf tied under the chin will accent the look of soft weak muscles and sag in the jowls.

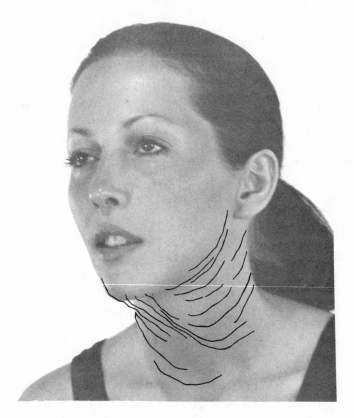

Vertical Neck Folds or Cords:
The Turkey Neck

DESCRIPTION

Sagging skin just under the chin and on the upper part of the neck makes any face look unattractive. "Turkey neck" is produced when the muscles lengthen and the skin over the muscles dries and sags.

PLAN

The muscles and skin on the neck are very sensitive. Have you noticed how the meat, or muscle tissue, on the neck of a chicken or turkey seems like a series of strings? Your neck is quite similar in construction. It is a bony column held together with muscles— flexible, strong, and graceful. As the muscles loosen and lengthen, the inner cords, invisible in the firm throat of youth, appear as vertical lines. The job is to tighten these muscles, strengthen them, and force moisture into the neck skin to reproduce the smooth column of a young neck.

Exercise will tighten and firm these muscles. Strangely, this sort of neck problem shows up more in a picture or photograph than in the mirror. Perhaps it is because the angle from which we usually see ourselves hides the under-chin and top neck area. However, if you see any sag at all when you look at your profile in the mirror, you doubtlessly have the beginning of a ''turkey neck.''

ERASINGS

Lubrication. Heavily cream your entire neck and shoulders. Cover the area by smoothing the cream upward from the collarbone to the chin. Don't forget the area under your earlobe.

Firming. You will notice that the cords fall in two folds, one at either side of the chin. This is because the bone in the center of the chin seems to support the center skin and flesh. The positioning of the teeth and neck are very important in these exercises:

Place your teeth on edge: position your teeth so that the top and bottom meet evenly, regardless of whether this is your natural bite.

Keep your mouth closed and try not to tense the side of your face or jaw. You will be able to tell if there is tension by an ache after you position your teeth.

Holding your teeth firmly in place, raise your chin toward the ceiling. Try to point your chin at a spot directly over your head. You will notice that this stretches and tenses the neck muscles as it tightens them.

Holding the position and pointing the chin, count slowly to ten. Relax. Repeat three times. After one week, increase to five times.

You will notice that your eyes close when you point your chin upward. This is natural. Try to keep your face as relaxed as possible. It is a temptation to practice this exercise at odd moments during the day, but beware of doing the exercise without first creaming your neck and shoulders.

Within a short period, your neck should feel stronger and more flexible.

Smoothing. Because of its sensitivity, neck skin often dries considerably before other skin on the face. For the smoothing, use a large heated soup spoon, or a silver ladle with rounded tip.

Hold the outer bowl of the soup spoon against the collarbone. With a pushing, smoothing motion, glide and guide the bowl up from the middle of the collarbones to the chin.

Repeat the smoothing motion from the collarbones and shoulders, up the neck, to the chin, first on one side of neck and then on the other (or, if desired, use two spoons or ladles and work on both sides of the neck simultaneously).

Be sure that the neck is kept lubricated up to the ears. Work the cream into the skin with the spoon, working up and out, up and out, from the middle of the neck to under the ears.

Do not forget the back of the neck. After creaming well, smooth the skin on the back of the neck by holding the large spoon by the handle. Work from shoulder to hairline.

Always work from the shoulders and base of the neck up to the chin and ears. Do not work *around* the neck; work in the direction in which the stringy cords form.

FREQUENCY

The neck muscles do not respond as well to exercise and smoothings as do many other muscles. It may be because gravity keeps fighting against the exercises. While you may not see immediate results from these exercises, you will notice that the skin of the neck will be smoother and softer, and will take on a satin glow, even after the first smoothing.

Don't be discouraged. After about two weeks the neck should firm noticeably, first directly under the chin, then down toward the neck column

CAMOUFLAGE

High collars, soft bows, and soft blouses often cover the neck or distract the eye from the sags in the neck. This is desirable not only because the skin is covered up, but because a soft silk scarf protects the sensitive skin on the neck from further damage. Avoid dangling earrings, or a hair style that is mid-neck in length. This only serves to attract attention to the least attractive part of the neck.

Always avoid busy patterns, bright or garish scarfs, glittery jewelry, or any other ornamentation that would attract attention to the neck. Pearls, a handsome gold chain, or a collarlike necklace that will sit more on the shoulders than clasp the neck will be more becoming.

Part Four

YOUR BODY

Ten

WHAT DO YOU REALLY LOOK LIKE?

Most of us don't know what we really look like, what impression we make when we walk into a party or meeting, when we're waiting to be seated at the theater or a restaurant, when we go into the supermarket or bank, when we're being interviewed for a job.

Here is how you can find out how you look to others.

1. Get a paper bag large enough to fit over your head.
2. Pull it over your head. Feel, with your fingers, where your eyes are and where your chin is. Mark with pen or pencil.
3. Take off the bag and cut off around the open end, *below* the mark for your chin.
4. Cut eye holes.
5. Pull down your window shades, blinds, or draperies and take off your clothes. All of them. Panties too.
6. Put the bag over your head again.
7. Now look at yourself—painful though you may find it to be. Examine your thighs. Notice if your buttocks sag. Look for wrinkles in the body, stretch marks, other problems.
8. Take out your body chart. On your body chart, which is for your personal and *private* use, mark down every wrinkle or other problem you see, including sagging tummy, sagging breasts, too-fat waist, lumpy thighs, sagging bottom.

Your body chart is your reminder of what you look like to *others* and of problems you want to free yourself from.

When you decide to improve your figure as well as face, a body chart or "body image map" is a real help. To create one, you need the aid of a friend, or a friendly husband. On the chart, you will mark your problems, indicate your goals, and keep a record of your progress toward those goals.

Besides your trusted "confederate," you need some heavy paper, such as shelving paper, wallpaper, or large sheets of newspaper, plus Scotch tape or paste.

1. Create a piece of paper that is your height and your width, plus six inches in the length and breadth.
2. Strip to your bra and panties, take off your shoes, and lie down on the paper.
3. Ask friend or husband to trace the outline of your body on the paper, using a grease pencil or marking pencil. It seems to work best if the crayon or large-sized marker is held rigid by being attached to a ruler or some sort of "pointer."
4. Stand up. Survey your shape on the body map you have just made.
5. Write down on the side of the map (or in your workbook) any and all problems you see.
   Now, your husband, friend, or lover willing, you might make a map of your confederate's body so that you can both work simultaneously on problem bulges and wrinkles.
6. You can keep the chart in your closet, hanging on a hanger, as a constant reminder of your goals and progress.
7. As you conquer each wrinkle on your torso and legs, you erase or mark out the spot on your chart. Those erasures provide a real feeling of satisfaction. (You might even mark each conquered wrinkle with a star—a continuing reminder of victories won.) Very good therapy for a poor ego.
8. If overweight is one of your challenges, note on your chart each time you lose three pounds. When you lose ten pounds, reward yourself with a gold star.

Eleven

CREATING A WRINKLE-FREE BODY

Are you afraid to appear on the beach without a tan? Do you feel soft, flabby, and wrinkled? Do you avoid looking at yourself in a mirror when you dress? There are ways of ridding the body of wrinkles. Just as the spoons are used to smooth away wrinkles on your face, a simple device can be used to smooth away wrinkles on the most commonly wrinkled parts of the body.

Chapters 12 to 17 provide a variety of body exercises that can be used at almost any time of the day. They range from the very traditional exercises to more unusual ones.

Any of the exercises can be used with the suggested smoothing techniques. The difference is that following the exercises, we suggest that you smooth away your body wrinkles with ordinary glass jars that are probably in your kitchen cabinets right now. Here is how:

Find a round wine or similar style bottle. It should have a smooth, firm, unridged surface.

Be sure you have a secure cork or screw type top that is leak-proof. Warm the bottle and fill it with about two cups of very hot water. Be careful that the glass is warm enough so it will not crack.

Cover your body with cream, body lotion, or a lubricant such as seed or vegetable oil.

Check your own body chart (Chapter 10), and decide on the ''target wrinkles.''

Hold the bottle firmly at the neck, either with one hand or in both hands.

Roll and press the bottle over the part of your body that you
want to smooth.
Roll and press at least 5 times. Relax; roll and press again.
Roll each wrinkle, smoothing each at least 10 times.

The following exercises are for specific body wrinkles—specific ways
for smoothing those wrinkles.

For Front of Neck, Chest and Breasts, Armpits, Diaphragm, Waist

Most people will prefer a long-necked wine bottle, for this exercise,
since the neck of the bottle makes it easier to control the ''roll.'' The
bottle shape also aids the exercise.

EXERCISE

For this exercise, fill the bottle with about two cups of hot water, then
cork or recap the bottle.
1. Hold the bottle by the neck.
2. Extend the right arm directly out from the body.
3. Hold the bottle by the neck. Swing the bottle to shoulder
   height, holding arm out from the side of your body, back
   down to side, again to shoulder height.
4. Repeat 10 times. Change arms and repeat with left arm.

SMOOTHING

1. Apply body lotion or cream to your body.
2. Hold the bottle in one hand.
3. Roll the bottle firmly across the opposite shoulder, around
   the side of the breast, under the armpit, and down to
   the waist.

4. Roll and press the bottle from the waist, over the diaphragm and *upward* on the breast. *(Do not roll down on the breast.)* Roll and press around the breast and up to the collarbone, further along the collarbone on to the neck to the jawline.
5. Place the bottle in the opposite hand and work the other side of your body, following directions 2 and 3.
6. Repeat until bottle cools.

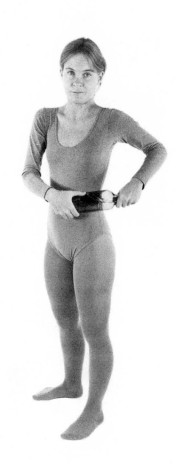

117

For Sides of Body, Under Arms, Down Sides of Legs, Back of Knees, Down to Ankles

We seldom see ourselves from the side—the view most others have of us.

Fill a large jar or wine bottle with about two cups of very hot water. Seal securely.

EXERCISE

A few minutes of general exercise—running in place, jumping rope, or general body bends and stretches—is helpful.

SMOOTHING

1. Cream or oil your body.
2. Hold the filled wine bottle by the neck, and roll the bottle down the side of the body, working on the same side as the hand that holds the bottle, or on the opposite side of the body.
3. Pay special attention to the knees, front and back, the lower limb, especially the back of the calf, and the ankles.

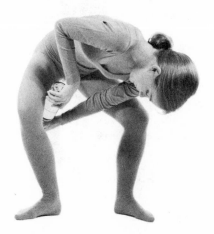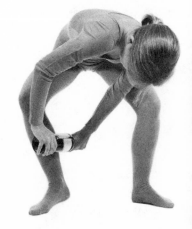

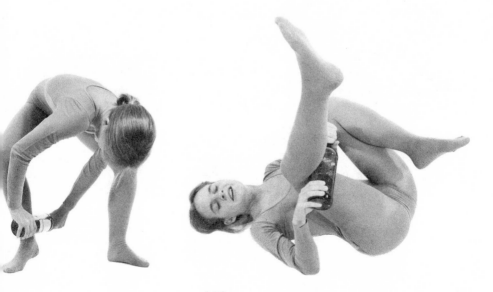

For Buttocks, Upper Thighs, Inner Thighs, ''Cellulite'' Area

This area is easy to reach with a long-necked wine bottle. Some people find the back of the thigh and the buttocks difficult to smooth with an ordinary jar.

Fill the bottle half full with very hot water.

EXERCISE

This exercise forces blood to flow from the legs to the body. You might follow it by running in place or jumping rope for a few minutes.

1. Lie on your back, legs held close together.
2. Do not bend your knees, but raise the legs so that they are at an angle to your body.
3. Open and close the legs, so that your legs work in a scissors motion. Try to hold the legs and knees stiff.
4. Repeat the leg exercise at least 3 times.

SMOOTHING

1. Cream or oil your body.
2. Hold the hot bottle or jar in both hands, and starting at the top of the thigh, roll bottle down the length of each leg from torso to knee.
3. Don't forget the inner thigh. Roll against the soft inner skin of the inside of the thigh.
4. Keep working down from the torso to the knees.
5. Roll up again from knees to torso.
6. Roll over the knee joint, gently.
7. Roll hard over the heavy muscle-fat deposits on the back of the thighs.

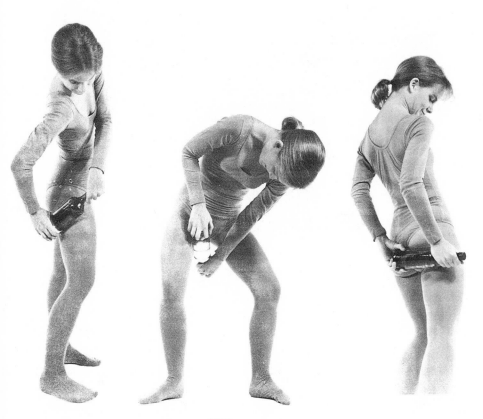

For Arms, Upper Arms and Shoulders, Inner Upper Arms, Outer Upper Arms and Fat Deposits, Rough Skin on Outer Upper Arms, Lower Arms and Dry Skin, Elbows

You are likely to prefer a small slender bottle for this rolling operation, but a long-necked wine bottle can also make a very good roller. You will have to use your right hand when working on your left arm, and your left hand when working on your right arm.

Fill two bottles with hot water, and be sure that the necks are tightly sealed. Hold the bottles by the necks.

EXERCISE

Holding one bottle in each hand, extend arms to the side. Try to hold your wrists stiff and keep the blood circulating through the entire length of the arm.

1. Using a rotating motion, swing the bottles in a figure "eight" motion.
2. Lift and circle with each arm extended from the shoulder. Repeat 10 times, then relax.

SMOOTHING

1. Oil or cream your arms and elbows.
2. Holding the neck of one bottle in your left hand, cross over the front of your body and roll the warm, water-filled bottle up the entire length of your right arm up and around the arm pit.
3. Stress the elbow and the area just over the elbow.
4. Work from the outside of the arm to the inside of the arm.
5. Repeat steps 2 through 4, 3 times, covering the entire arm.
6. Now repeat with the bottle in the right hand, working on the left arm.

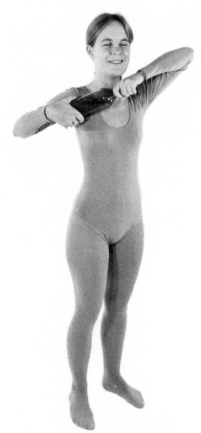

For Elbows and Wrists, Inner Elbows, Outer Elbows, Inner Wrists, Outer Wrists

You might prefer a small, slender bottle for this smoothing. However, the trusty long-necked wine bottle will do well here, too. This time, however, the *neck* should be used for smoothing the area around the wrists.

Fill two bottles with two cups of water each.

EXERCISE

1. Holding a bottle in each hand, flex the arms at the elbows so that the bottles cross over the front of the chest.
2. Draw bottles back, with the elbows still bent.
3. Swing bottles over the chest to a cross-armed position. Don't let them crash!
4. Repeat 10 times.

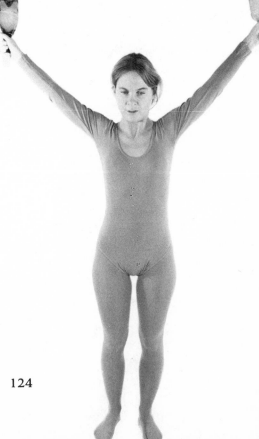

124

5. Hold the bottles by the necks, upside down. With arms bent at the elbows, hold the arms as close to the body as possible. The bottles should each stick up next to the ears with the bottoms toward the face.
6. Bending only the wrists, tip the bottles forward, one at a time, as far as you can while still keeping your elbows bent. This will strengthen the wrists and bring circulation to the hands and wrists.

SMOOTHING

1. Cream the hands, arms, and elbows well.
2. Roll the hands, arms, and elbows with the wine bottles, starting at the backs of the hands.
3. Work on your right hand while holding the wine bottle in the left hand.
4. Repeat by working on the left hand with bottle held in right.

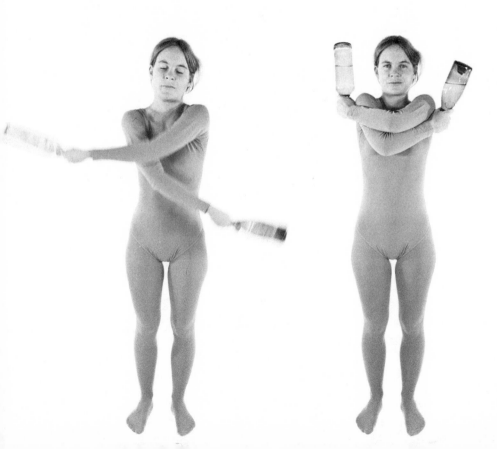

For Hands, Back of Hands, Palms, Thumbs, Nails, Wrists

The expression "beautiful right down to her fingertips," expresses the importance of your hands to your overall beauty. Your hands are as expressive as your face—and are almost as much in view. Soft, flexible hands are graceful and youthful. Here are some ways to create a "finger gymnasium" for your hands.

SMOOTHING

1. Select a jar with a large diameter. (You may also want to use several small jars, those that olives are packed in are perfect: tall, slim, and with a secure lid.) Fill the jar with two or more cups of hot water.
2. Cover the hands, wrists, and the lower part of the forearm with a heavy coat of moisturizer, cream, or polyunsaturate oil.
3. Place a towel over your lap. On the towel, place the large jar filled with water. It will be your work area.
4. Holding the large jar securely on your lap, rub your hands over the smoothing jar—back side down, palms up.
5. Place the thumbs so that they can roll directly against the smooth side of the jar. Roll back and forth, at least 10 times.
6. Holding your palms up, place the sides of the wrists against the jar and roll the wrists up and down against the jar.
7. Holding in your right hand an olive jar which you have filled with hot water, roll the jar, from fingertip to joint, inside and outside of each finger of your left hand.
8. Roll the jar around the nail area too.
9. Repeat on the right hand with the jar held in the left.

126

The dozens of body-language books that describe the observations of psychologists and sociologists describe the rise of hand gestures to convey conscious or unconscious feelings or motivations. The caressing gesture with graceful, long, flexible fingers has an obvious seductive message.

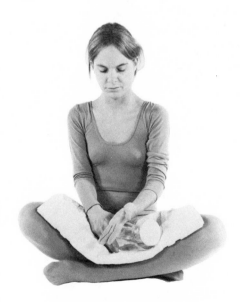

Part Five

EXERCISES

Twelve

EXERCISE: SHOULD YOU STAND UP, RUN OR LIE DOWN?

All exercise is good, if it is within the framework of practicality and your own capabilities and inclination. How and where you exercise is really up to you, but it is never practical to exercise beyond the point of fatigue. There is a lot to commend exercising lying down, flat on the bed or floor, or on a slant board. The floor, bed, or board supports you as you work, taking the strain from the body. Also, gravity will be working with you instead of against you. When you stand, you must align and balance your body because gravity is pulling you down, causing your organs to sink. When you lie down, the abdomen drops back toward the spine; the force of gravity holds you flat on the floor.

In this section you will find exercises to help you wake up easily; exercises to do in or on the bed or floor or slant board; exercises to do in the bath, for eyes, mouth, throat, ankles, feet; exercises to do sitting up, some to do while watching TV; stretching exercises; desk exercises; exercises to do while telephoning; exercises to do while washing dishes or cleaning your teeth. This idea is to put your time to the most effective use for the sake of your health and beauty. Encourage time to serve more than one of your goals simultaneously. Many people think that exercising is boring—these exercises should overcome that objection because they are done at odd moments and while you are waiting for something else.

Exercise Questionnaire

Read over the questionnaire below. You should be getting at least 10 minutes of exercise daily. If you don't engage in daily exercise, you might want to make it one of your beauty goals. Exercising results in firm muscles, good circulation and a glowing skin. It also acts as a stimulant to many people, and they find they not only look better but are more alert.

Place a piece of paper next to the lists if you don't want to write directly in your book.

Section I

Do you follow and organized program that includes any of the following sports:	Usually	Sometimes	Never
calisthenics	_____	_____	_____
yoga	_____	_____	_____
ballet dancing	_____	_____	_____
tap dancing	_____	_____	_____
modern dancing	_____	_____	_____
ballroom dancing	_____	_____	_____
fencing	_____	_____	_____
swimming	_____	_____	_____
skipping rope	_____	_____	_____
jogging	_____	_____	_____
tennis	_____	_____	_____
golf	_____	_____	_____
walking	_____	_____	_____
bowling	_____	_____	_____
volley ball	_____	_____	_____
active play with children	_____	_____	_____
gardening	_____	_____	_____
softball	_____	_____	_____
basketball	_____	_____	_____
ice skating	_____	_____	_____
roller skating	_____	_____	_____
bicycle riding	_____	_____	_____

Section II

The questions in this section are very open. The idea is to alert you to exactly how much exercise you are getting every day. You may be getting enough . . . without any program. And you may not be getting enough, even if you do participate in a specific sport. A minimum of 10 minutes a day is considered essential by many experts.

Do you usually exercise: less than one hour a day   _____

                   less than 30 minutes a day   _____

                   less than three hours a week   _____

                   not at all   _____

Do you usually exercise for: weight loss   _____

                     muscle tone   _____

                     specific medical reasons   _____

                     because it is fun   _____

Section III

Do you have a favorite physical exercise that is not mentioned in our list? If so, what is it?

If you exercise for less than 20 minutes daily, we suggest you write on your questionnaire how long you do exercise, and how much time you actually spend in physical activity. As stated, the minimum might be 10 minutes a day; but you might feel and look better if you try to work up to a consistent pattern of 20 minutes a day.

Thirteen

EXERCISES TO DO LYING DOWN

STRENGTHENING AND TRIMMING LOWER ABDOMEN

Situated on the sides and front of the abdomen are broad, flat, thin muscles which brace and support the lower part of the abdomen. With age and inactivity, these muscles relax and weaken, producing that unattractive condition called pot belly, all too frequently evident in men over 50 and too readily displayed by women of ''un certain'' age when they wear slacks.

From these broad, thin muscles, other external muscles proceed in various directions. These muscles overlap and interlace, forming a webbing designed to support and protect the underlying bowels and organs. These external muscles are braced by a system of deep-seated internal muscles, further protection for the inner organs.

The exercises that follow firm the abdomen, sometimes the abdomen and back, sometimes abdomen and buttocks, sometimes abdomen and thighs.

ABDOMEN EXERCISE

This exercise will strengthen and flatten the abdomen. It's a great aid for constipation too.

1. Lie on your back on a bed or floor.
2. Bend right leg upward and inward until foot touches left leg above knee and right knee is bent over and beyond the upper left leg.

135

3. While bending right leg and knee, draw right hip up, toward the waist.
4. Relax right leg to outstretched position.
5. Repeat with left leg and hip.
6. Alternate exercises for a total of 3 times for each side.
7. As you become accustomed to exercise, increase up to a total of 10 times for each side.

WHOLE BODY EXERCISE

The benefits of this exercise are improved circulation and improved skin tone.

1. Lie on your right side, on the floor or bed.
2. Fold arms over stomach and grasp elbows with hands.
3. Throw your head back as far as you can, at the same time stretching your body and legs to the fullest possible length.
4. Exert pressure upon your elbows with your hands while, simultaneously, you stretch and tense your body into rigidity. (In the beginning, only exert half-pressure on elbows.)
5. Hold for *slow* count of 10.
6. Relax effort during a slow count of 5.
7. Repeat.
8. Turn to left side and repeat alternate tensing–relaxing movement, 2 times.
9. This is a strenuous exercise designed to speed the flow of blood throughout the body. As you gain strength through the exercise, you can increase the pressure on your elbows and increase the number of repeats to a maximum of 5 exercises on each side.

TORSO TRIMMER

This exercise strengthens stomach and side muscles.

1. Lie on your right side on the floor or bed.
2. Simultaneously, lift head and legs as high as you can while balancing yourself with opposite hand and arm.
3. Repeat twice.

136

4. Shift to left side
5. Repeat exercise twice.
6. After two weeks, increase to 3 lifts for each side.

THE NECK

Two large muscles attached to the base of the skull descend to the shoulders as the principal supports of the neck. Another pair of large muscles, attached to the skull immediately behind the ears and descending to the collarbone, brace the sides of the neck. Minor muscles moving in a variety of directions contribute support. Muscles of the neck are voluntary and can be exercised at will to increase their size, strength, and elasticity.

The large muscle attached to the thyroid bone (in men this is called the Adam's Apple) ascends to attach to the lower part of the chin bone.

Unless exercised, the muscle withers and atrophies so that the full round throat of youth develops hollows, seams, lines, and, in time, a crepey look, often with loose hanging jowls and folds called dewlaps.

NECK EXERCISE #1

This exercise is to improve throat contours, diminish wrinkles, and decrease nervous tension.

1. Lie on your right side on a bed or floor.
2. Place your right thumb, *firmly*, under the chin, or about the center of the large muscle which extends from the Adam's apple to chin.
3. Exert upward pressure with the thumb.
4. Throw your head back as far as it will go. Note tension in neck muscles.
5. Keeping your thumb on your chin, bring head forward until chin touches chest. This relaxes tension.
6. Repeat 10 times.
7. Turn to left side, put your left thumb under the chin, and repeat 10 times.
8. After one week increase the exercise as desired, up to 30 times, or as your time will allow.

137

NECK EXERCISE #2

The following exercise strengthens the muscles along the sides of the neck, diminishes wrinkles, and enlarges the throat.

1. Lie on your right side on the floor or bed.
2. Interlock arms over the diaphragm.
3. Turn your head left to touch your chin on top of the shoulder.
4. Return chin to center front.
5. Repeat 5 times.
6. Turn to the left side.
7. Repeat exercise 5 times, turning the chin right to the shoulder top.

Fourteen

EXERCISES TO DO STANDING UP

FOR LUNGS, KNEES, AND LEGS

This double-duty exercise combines deep breathing with a standard preseason exercise for skiers: knee bends, plus arm swings.

The benefits are greater lung capacity and greater leg flexibility.

1. Stand outdoors, or in front of open window, feet slightly apart, arms on hips.
2. Inhale deeply, expanding lower rib cage and abdomen, as you swing your arms wide to shoulder height and then upward until your arms are perpendicular to your body.
3. As you exhale slowly, hold your torso erect and bend your knees. (You may find them stiff at first, but they'll limber up as you continue the exercise on a daily basis or more often.)
4. Repeat 5 times to start, if you have not been exercising much. Increase the number until you are doing the exercise 20 times a day.

FOR NECK AND THYROID

Muscles are exercised from chest to mouth and lower cheek in this exercise.

While some believe a well-functioning liver is the key to forestalling visible aging, others believe that the secret lies in the thyroid.

The thyroid, as well as other organs, benefits from exercise. Do this exercise alone, or only in the presence of an understanding companion.

1. Stand erect, head centered, shoulders back.
2. Stick out tongue—farther—farther—farther!
3. Stretch and hold.
4. Relax.
5. Repeat 5 to 10 times.

EYE EXERCISE

This eye exercise will improve circulation and diminish wrinkles.

1. Stand erect. Try not to move your head.
2. Roll eyes up, look at ceiling.
3. Look at your feet.
4. Look left as far as possible.
5. Look right as far as possible.
6. Repeat, alternately from side to side, 10 times.
7. Blink eyes rapidly for 60 seconds.

FOR BODY FLEXIBILITY

As you become adept in this exercise, which is to be done as rapidly as possible, you'll find you're catching more buses!

1. Stand with your left side to a wall, near enough so that you can touch it easily with your outspread hand. Your feet should be 18 to 24 inches apart.
2. Rapidly touch the wall with your left hand as high as you can reach, and then bending at the waist on a downward swing with the same hand, touch the toes of your right foot.
3. Repeat rapidly 5 times.
4. Turn around and repeat the exercise touching your right hand to the wall and then to the left foot.
5. Repeat, alternating, for a total of 10 times.

Fifteen

❧EXERCISES TO DO IN MOTION❧

The easiest exercise for most people to do is walking. Walking can be undertaken even by the overweight. However, if your feet hurt, you may not think that it's so easy. If they do hurt, you might consult a podiatrist to find out why you have a foot problem, and try to remove the cause. It is a rare problem that can't be solved. Perhaps you should consider wearing a different kind of shoe. Many women have never worn sandals or sneakers; they can be a joy for your feet. Shoes should be changed more than once a day. Often, the solution is to put an end to smoking: the relationship between aching feet and cigarettes appears to be the adverse effect heavy smoking has on the circulation.

Dancing is also a good exercise for anyone. If you don't have anyone to dance with, put on the music and dance by yourself. Or join a dance class—ballroom, ballet—or any other kind. You will develop suppleness of body and strengthen your muscles and the bones of your feet too. Dancer-comedian Ray Bolger continues to dance two hours daily and, in his seventies, moves with the grace and ease he displayed when he was twenty.

Running is an extraordinary exercise, and so are jogging and skipping rope. It is best to run and jog and skip rope on the grass or ground, not on hard wood or pavement. You can skip rope and even run in place indoors, but it is preferable to do so on a mat so that there isn't the body shock of landing on a hardwood floor.

Skating and downhill or cross-country skiing are wonderful exercises for people of any age. The best exercise of all is swimming. It provides benefits for almost anyone. Medical studies have shown that swimming can even cure some asthmatics. If you can't swim, just get into a pool, hang on to the side, and kick. You'll find it easier to exercise under water, and if exercising is new to you, start with a few simple poolside exercises, plus the exercises you do in bed.

Sixteen

ANYTIME ALMOST ANYWHERE EXERCISES

Lack of time is the most common excuse for not exercising. Yet exercise can take as much time as you choose. If you put your mind to it, you can find a lot of time to exercise—while doing something else. For instance:

1. *Standing on a street corner waiting for a bus, wearing flat-heeled shoes:* Rock back on your heels, forward on your toes. Repeat at will. (If other people look at you curiously, smile blandly and say nothing, or if you choose, state lightly, ''Exercising.'')

2. *Riding in a bus or car:* Pull in your abdomen; contract your buttocks. Relax. Repeat at will. (Note: the exercise can be done in a car by a *passenger, never* by the driver, even while waiting at a red light.)

3. *Riding in an elevator:*
   a. Bus exercise (i.e., same as #1 above).
   b. Dove exercise. Turn head to left, touching chin to shoulder. Return to center. Turn head to right and touch chin to shoulder. (Don't be self-conscious about the other elevator passengers; they're not likely even to notice you. Try it and you'll see.)

4. *Sitting in a movie theater or in front of a TV set:*
   a. Bus exercise.
   b. Ankle rolls. Try to make your soles touch by pivoting your feet.

c. "Prayer" exercise, to strengthen fingers, hands, and arm muscles: press hands against each other, with as much force as you can muster. Relax. Repeat at will.

d. Exercise the liver by massaging as deeply as possible, firmly pressing your fists against the right side of your body, slightly above the waist.

5. *Doing dishes, cleaning vegetables, cooking:* Stand in stocking or bare feet on a "spiky" rubber foot-exerciser mat. If your feet aren't tough enough at first, spread a towel over the "spikes." The mat stimulates circulation and, it's claimed, provides other benefits.

6. *Waiting for someone to answer the telephone:* Blow up a balloon. This is a good exercise for your lungs, the muscles of your mouth and cheeks, and all of you, since your health and beauty depend upon adequate oxygen intake and dispersal of poisonous waste. We find it helpful to keep a balloon by each telephone and to carry a packet too. Do this exercise as often as possible. Five minutes a day is good to start, working up to 15 minutes a day. If more than one member of your family does the balloon-blowing exercise, buy different colored balloons and assign a specific color to each person. This will ensure that you each have your own personal balloons.

These are just to get you started *thinking* about where and when you can exercise. You can make time serve a double purpose.

Seventeen

🌿WAKE-UP EXERCISES TO DO IN BED🌿

These exercises are to be done lying flat in bed, on a firm mattress, with no pillow beneath your head. It is a healthy, delightful way to make the bridge between sleep and morning activity.

ANKLE ROTATION

1. Rotate both feet so toes point out.
2. Repeat 10 times.
3. Rotate both feet so toes point in.
4. Repeat 10 times.

THE ROCKER

1. Thrust legs straight out, heels against the mattress, and pull toes back toward you until a hard stretch is felt throughout the feet and legs.
2. Rock toes forward as far as they will go.
3. Relax.
4. Repeat a minimum of 5 times and as many more as you enjoy. Once you start doing this exercise, you may be reluctant to stop even at 20.

LEG KICK

1. Raise right knee, then kick leg straight out, ending with heel flat against mattress, toes up.
2. Relax.

3. Kick left leg forward, hard.
4. Relax.
5. Repeat, alternating legs, for a minimum of 10 times each leg. This is an exercise you should do fast as well as hard. You'll feel muscle involvement throughout your legs and buttocks and into your waist.

THE DOVE

1. Lying on back, keep shoulders level and turn head to the right until chin rests on shoulder. (You may not be able to do this in the beginning. Persist. It's worth it.)
2. Return head to center.
3. Repeat to left.
4. Repeat twice more, or as many times as you choose.

NECK STRETCH WITH DEEP BREATHING

1. While inhaling deeply, lower your head until chin rests on chest. Hold for count of 3.
2. While exhaling slowly, raise head and stretch neck backward until the crown of your head rests on the mattress. Hold for count of 3.
3. Repeat 3 times.

SCALP AWAKENER

1. Place fingers of both hands on scalp, heels of the palms at the temples.
2. Press scalp back with palms of hands while exercising scalp with fingertips.
3. Repeat 10 times.
4. Shift fingers to different part of the scalp, to exercise the entire head.
5. Complete exercise by placing fingertips on either side of nape of neck.
6. Rotate in circular motion.

146

LUNG AWAKENER

1. Place palms of hands at lower rib cage.
2. Breathe in through nose, feeling ribs expand and abdomen extend.
3. Breathe out through nose, firmly forcing air out from all areas of the lungs, including the normally neglected bottom of the lungs, by pressing palms of hands firmly against the rib cage.
4. Repeat 5 times initially, gradually working up to 10 times.

EAGLE'S FLIGHT

1. Put tips of fingers on each shoulder, holding them there throughout the exercise.
2. Rotate shoulders back, and circle shoulders rapidly for a minimum of 10 times.

BODY STRETCH

1. Put heels against mattress, toes up.
2. Bend elbows over head.
3. Stretch body as much as possible, thrusting both legs forward and stretching neck upward, along the mattress as far as possible.
4. Repeat 10 times.

TUMMY TRIMMER

1. Lie on your back, legs straight, arms raised straight up, perpendicular to the body.
2. Slowly sit up.
3. Repeat six times.

GETTING IT TOGETHER

1. Lie on back, knees bent, feet together, soles flat against the bed, arms extended at sides, palms down.
2. Draw right knee toward chest while raising left arm up and back until it extends straight with shoulder.

3. Draw left knee toward chest while raising right arm up and back.
4. With knees raised toward chest and arms extended, inhale deeply.
5. Exhale while you raise right leg perpendicular to the torso while left arm falls until left hand rests on right leg.
6. Lower legs and arms to original position.
7. Repeat, starting with left leg and right arm.
8. Repeat 5 times, alternating from left to right.

EYE OPENER

1. Open eyes wide, keeping head flat against mattress. Look straight up at the ceiling.
2. Roll eyes slowly left as far as they can go to the corner of the ceiling.
3. Follow ceiling slowly around the room until eyes return to starting point.
4. Repeat 10 times.
5. Repeat to the right for 10 slow eye sweeps.
6. Squeeze eyes shut.
7. Stretch eyes wide.
8. Repeat 10 times for a wide-awake start of the day.

Part Six

THE
ANTI-WRINKLE
CAMPAIGN

Eighteen

ANTI-WRINKLE WAYS TO CLEAN YOUR FACE, FACE THE WORLD, AND GO TO BED

Use soap and water to clean your face at least twice a day, morning and night. You cannot wash your face too often; even ten times a day is fine. But you *can* use soap too often. Restrict its use to twice a day as a rule; it can be increased to three, four, or even five times a day if the occasion calls for it: if you are in a particularly polluted atmosphere; if you're doing a dirty job; if you're wearing heavy makeup which must be cleaned off before new makeup can be applied, or before going to sleep.

Cleansing cream? We advise against it. It doesn't clean as easily and thoroughly as soap.

The kind of soap you use is most important. The fact that it's white or claims to be pure doesn't mean it's good for your skin. A great many soaps on the market are merely lye, fat, and perfume. We recommend nonperfumed soap because many people are unknowingly allergic to perfume. There are many good soaps on the market, clear and nonclear. Read the ingredients! In the Appendix is a list of some soaps we like.

151

1. Fill the basin with cool-to-warm water, as you prefer.
2. Wet your face.
3. Lather soap in your hands.
4. Apply to your face with the palms of your hands in upward—always upward—motions. Press the soap on firmly, even massage in lightly. Don't scrub!
   You can use a natural facial sponge if you prefer. But if you do use a sponge, wash it in *very hot* water afterwards. If the water in your faucet isn't too hot for your hands, drop your sponge into a pot of boiling water for a few minutes.
   If you want to use a washcloth, do so. But use it only once! Bacteria collect on washcloths, and many people put germs on their faces from their washcloths. It's really deplorable that many people use the same washcloth for a whole week. It should be used for only a *single wash*. No more. Hands are easier to use, and you can't possibly hurt you face with the palms of your hands—when you wash *up!*
5. Rinse. Not once. A minimum of 25 times. Fifty times is better. It doesn't take long. Even one wash with soap plus 50 rinses will make your skin feel softer and finer, and within ten days you will certainly see a decided improvement.
   Rinse up! You can *splash* water on your face and neck (wear a shower cap if you want to keep your hair dry), or you can *press* it on. We prefer to slap-press the rinse water in upward motions: three upward, pressing slaps normally use up a palmful of water.
   Don't forget the neck. That requires the same number of rinses.
   Count the rinses. How else will you know when you reach 50? The objective is to rid your skin of every last smidgeon of soap.
6. Pat/press your skin dry with a medium-weight terry towel, preferably white. Dark-colored and bright-colored towels, even from the best manufacturers, too often run.

You don't want dye on your clean face! And, some people have a slightly allergic reaction to the dye in fabrics.

7. Restore the normal acid balance of your face. Splash on water diluted with lemon juice— ¼ to ½ lemon to one pint of water (preferably spring water). Spraying your face with the lemon rinse is better—ten rinses for each side of your face. Spray your throat and neck too (and bosom if you want to). You can use a spray such as is used to spray plants. (Choose a glass jar. A plastic jar is all right when you're traveling, but on a daily basis you don't want to take chances of chemicals from the plastic leaking into your good lemon water.) You can use an empty Windex bottle for the same purpose. Just boil it well before you use it!

8. Apply an herbal-rich moisturizer right on top of the wet skin. (Make sure it contains no mineral oil.) The water on your face forms a bond with the moisturizers so that the goodies in the moisturizer penetrate the pores to provide the greatest benefit for your skin.

Don't dip your fingers into the jar. Take out a small amount with a spatula and put it onto a small clean plate or piece of waxed paper. Don't use foil. The purpose of keeping your fingers out of the jar is to prevent contamination.

Apply the moisturizer to your face in large, upward, outward circular motions over your cheeks, temples, and forehead. Apply to the nose area in smaller, upward, outward circles, and between the eyes in a circular motion. Gently finger-press around the eye, starting from the nose for both the eyelid and under the eye. (We are assuming that the moisturizer you use will be both herbal-rich and light in texture.) Avoid heavy creams on your face at all times and particularly avoid those traditional eye creams that are heavy, like petroleum jelly, and are likely to pull the skin. An eye cream formulated especially for wearers of soft contact lenses is referred to in the Resource List of the Appendix.

There are additional options to consider for the day. If you

want to give your skin extra nutrients, you may choose to
top the moisturizer with a cellular cream which contains
soluble collagen protein in a light creamy base of sesame
oil and possibly cocoa butter, beeswax, and such skin-kind
vitamins as A, D, E, and F. (See Resource List.)

9. Whenever you wash your face with soap during the day,
follow with the 25 to 50 rinses, the lemon-water spray
(or you can use water with apple cider vinegar), and
moisturizer.

10. If your face feels oily during the day, and it's likely to,
put a clean linen square (handkerchief) over your face,
press the handkerchief against your face to soak up the oil,
and then wash with warm water followed by tepid,
followed with the moisturizer on your wet face. If you
have an excessive amount of oil, or a troubled skin, you
will want a soap-and-water cleansing three times a day or
even more, plus the pH balancing rinses and the plain
water facial baths and moisturizer.

You will soon find it a special joy when you feel able to
face the world free of makeup, or with only a minimum.

BEFORE BED

Whether you wear makeup or not, always cleanse your face, throat,
and neck before you go to bed. Repeat the soaping/rinsing procedure
of the morning. If you are going to do a selection of facial exercises
and smoothings, proceed as follows:

1. Let your face air dry.
2. With your clean, dry face, perform the facial exercises of
your choice.
3. Spray your face with the lemon or vinegar rinse.
4. Apply your favorite moisturizer.
5. Allow to absorb five minutes while you prepare your
''beauty table,'' including boiling water and silver
spoons, for your smoothings.
6. Apply your favorite cream or oil, using the upward,
outward circular motions on face, throat, and neck.
7. Perform the facial and body smoothings of your choice
And so to bed—to dream of beauty.

WEEKLY

Once a week exfoliate your skin, by ridding it of dead skin. Exfoliating can be aided by a cream of your choice or juice of a favorite exfoliating fruit, either papaya or pineapple.

1. Apply cream or fruit in upward, outward circular motions on the face, throat, neck, and backs of hands. Chest too, if you wish.
2. Allow cream to dry two or three minutes (five for pineapple juice).
3. Holding the skin firm with one hand, rub the first two fingers of the other hand back and forth, up and down, over the portion of the skin held firmly. It is essential that you hold the skin firmly so that the back-and-forth motion won't stretch it.
4. When you have gone over the entire surface of the skin, rinse the skin and apply moisturizer on the wet skin.

On a day or evening when you are not exfoliating your skin with cream or fruit, give yourself a weekly facial. Recipes for a variety of masques are contained in the Appendix and in Chapter 21: egg white alone; parsley–egg white–papaya–slippery elm; egg white and Milk of Magnesia; egg white and honey; clay, and fruit masques.

Use a commercial masque if you have a favorite but avoid like the plague "peel-off masks." They stretch the skin and encourage wrinkles.

Apply the mask, put absorbent cotton pads soaked in chilled witch hazel on your eyes, or, if your eyes are puffy, pads soaked in fresh potato juice, made by grating a raw potato, turn on soothing music, and lie down on your bed, mat, floor, or slant board and think beautiful thoughts for 20 or 30 minutes. Don't answer the phone. Don't talk to anyone. This is your time for beauty—and privacy.

MONTHLY

Once a month, or before any special occasion, consider giving yourself, or, better, having someone give you, a "mummy masque."

This is a masque that a certain famous spa charges $150 for. It's used by movie stars. We heard of one great Parisian beauty who

155

had given herself a mummy masque every night. She slept with it all night—apparently alone. She died in her late eighties absolutely wrinkle free. We think Ninon de Lenclos had more fun—while keeping wrinkle free with simple exercises performed in privacy. We think you'll have more fun too using the program offered in this book. Directions for the mummy masque appear in the Appendix.

Nineteen

ANTI-WRINKLE WAYS TO MAKE UP

In the Twenties, Thirties, and Forties, makeup was applied heavily to create artificial effects that popularized the film greats: Clara Bow of the cupid's bow mouth; Joan Crawford of the exaggerated lips; Marlene Dietrich of the bird's flight brows. Lipstick was dark and red and heavy, and so was nail polish.

The Sixties introduced the natural look which, despite the occasional flare-up of fads, has continued and intensified. It's part of the youth-generated demand for truth and honesty and being one's self. And the result? A lovelier, younger-looking world. Heavy, artificial makeup is definitely aging.

The natural look requires a cleaner, smoother, skin; squeaky clean hair; and clean nails. (Astonishing how really nice women can allow dirt to hide under their dark polish.)

While heavy makeup foundations rarely hid blemishes it did accentuate wrinkles—the makeup getting into folds and forming dark shadows to exaggerate the look of age—the wearers. Beguiled by persuasive advertising, believed they were presenting a beautiful mask to the world. In truth, the masks were rarely beautiful, and those who did look beautiful with the mask would have looked lovelier without it.

Makeup of the Seventies is lighter, less likely to sink into wrinkles to exaggerate them. Even so, care should be taken that the tone is right for the skin. A too pale or too dark, too pink or too yellow makeup foundation can make the wearer look sick or at least unhealthy and will accentuate rather than diminish lines.

A black woman has a particularly hard time finding a shade that complements her special shade of Black, since there are so many tones. Often she must mix her own. That sometimes is necessary too for Orientals, whose skin can range from pure ivory to bisque to "yellow-like" to brown, and some Caucasian women also take pleasure in mixing their own shades. If the shade used is too dark, the skin can look dirty—the antithesis of glowing. If the shade is too light, the effect can be ashy.

Use a good light when you are making up. If you must do it under electric light even by day, check your makeup with a hand mirror by a window before going out to face the world. Women who have passed three score and ten are the ones most likely to appear in the daylight with too much rouge and powder. The effect is pathetic. And that misfortune can happen to anyone who doesn't check with a hand mirror in the light of day. Nighttime and electricity call for deeper makeup since the electric light "washes out" color.

There are four contemporary approaches to facing the world with confidence:

1. Your naked face, dressed only with moisturizer, or moisturizer plus protein cream, or, when you're going to be in the sun, moisturizer plus sun screen or sun block, according to whether you want to obtain a tan or prevent one. And, tan-prevention is the best look for an over-30 face.)
2. The above, plus lipstick and/or eye makeup.
3. Makeup complete with foundation but without eye makeup.
4. Complete makeup, including the eyes.

Any one of these approaches is *right*. The choice is yours. And sometimes you'll want to vary your approach from naked-natural to complete makeup, depending upon the occasion, your costume, and your mood. For example, a complete makeup is as inappropriate for a day at the beach or camping as a mink stole. Both are dated.

FOUNDATIONS

Most foundations are a creamy liquid, and some contain moisturizing elements. The latter are recommended.

Don't select the color by matching the skin of the back of your hand. That's a different kind of skin—thinner, and usually a different color. You need to try out the foundation on your face.

There are pancake foundations too. These formerly were popular, but generally they are too heavy for a contemporary look and they seem to "sit" on top of the skin rather than appear to be part of the skin as a moisturizing liquid is supposed to do. A pancake makeup is likely to accentuate lines.

POWDER

Powder is back. Choose a color to match your foundation, or translucent is a good choice. Don't use a powder puff—not even a pretty swansdown. They inevitably harbor bacteria. Each time you powder, use a fresh ball of cotton. Then discard it. Put the powder on as thickly as you wish; then brush off the excess with a soft, natural bristle brush. The objective is to provide a matte finish.

LIPSTICK

A "wardrobe" of lipsticks is needed, so that you can vary the color with your costume or your mood. Sometimes you'll want to use two, a darker over a lighter, or a lighter over darker. Only the very young should use a pure bright red or a dark red, although black women may use plum or raspberry with great effectiveness. The paler, more natural shades are more flattering to anyone who is past the 40 point. They make a person look younger. Be sure the lipstick is nondrying in effect.

LIP GLOSS

Lip gloss can be worn over or instead of lipstick. It's lighter than lipstick in color and weight, yet provides moisturizing protection against adverse effects of sun, wind, air conditioning, and steam heat.

ROUGE

Rouge, or a blusher, or a bronzing gel can be a delightful addition, brushed lightly over the cheekbones. Some come in powder form, some in a tube, some in a stick, or in a small, moist or dry cake. Powder or cake rouge is used on *top* of powder, the creams and gels *under* powder. Use a light hand. The effect to be sought is the flush of healthy blood surging to the surface. Apply the color upward and outward from the bony protuberances directly beneath the outer corner of the eyes. Blend the color toward the temples.

EYE SHADOW

Like rouge, eye shadow is available in cream, powder, or cake. A powder eye shadow is particularly good for a skin that is inclined to be oily. Powder or cake can make the eyelid of an older person appear crepey, so cream-based colors are often a better choice. You may favor a single color, or two, and use those with every costume, or you may want to vary the colors with your costumes.

Blend from the inner corners of the lid and sweep across and up. Avoid applying color too close to the nose, especially if your eyes are set close together.

If you feel your eyes are ''too prominent,'' apply a deep-tone matte eye shadow, such as brown, on the lid. Apply a lighter shade of the same color on the bone between lid and brow, blending this right up to the brown brow.

If your eyes are wide apart but somewhat narrow and slit-like in shape you will want to experiment seeking a wide-open look. For a start, you might blend a light beige shadow between the inner corner of the eye and the bridge of the nose, and use this same pale tone at the outer corners of the eyes. On the eyelid itself, smooth on a deeper beige matte shadow or very light blue, light green, or pale lilac. On the bony section between lids and brows, use a medium hue of eye shadow, intensifying the color slightly at the outer corner of the eyes, to carry the eye of the beholder upward.

EYELINER

Start your eyeliner one-quarter of an inch from the inner corner of the eye, applying it in a very thin line close to the lashes and gradually lifting the line above the lashes as you move to the outer end of the lid. Extend the eyeliner one-eighth inch beyond the end of the lid, with a slight upward slant. The objective is to create a subtle upward look.

160

Take care not to stretch the skin of the eyelid when applying either eyeliner or eye shadow. This is not only bad for the skin but will cause a wrinkled, crepey look. If you can't put on eyeliner or eye shadow without stretching the lid, we earnestly urge that you forego these items. They will be the antithesis of beauty *aids* for you. If the lid is at all wrinkled, don't use eye powder or eyeliner. If you wish, use a creamy eye shadow. But we don't know of any eyeliner that won't cause wrinkled eyelids to look anything but more wrinkled.

EYEBROW PENCIL

Tweeze out any stray hairs from under the eyebrows. If you have long, straggly hairs in your brows, cut them short with cuticle scissors. If your brows are thin, you can apply eyebrow pencil in tiny, feather-like strokes, ending the brow with a slight up-flick.

Avoid the trap many older women fall into of shaping the brow *around* the eye, so that sometimes the brow ends at about the end of the eye. If your eyebrows naturally droop down, assiduously practice the exercise to lift them, and tweeze off the lower hairs to avoid the ''drooping'' look.

Some women find that eyebrow powder is more becoming than a pencil. Eyebrow powder usually works best for the person who likes rather thick brows. The technique is the same: tiny, feathery strokes. And the effect can be flattering for a 20-year-old or for a lady of 80 if she has strong features and personality. It is not for the porcelain lady of any age.

ARTIFICIAL LASHES

Artifical lashes, which originated in the Orient long ago, can be flattering and conducive to a bright, young look, or they can be disastrous. The effect depends less upon age or shape of eye than on the choice of lash. There are many kinds and shapes, and care should be taken that the lashes aren't exaggeratedly long. That may be an amusing look of artificiality upon someone very young, on a special occasion, but it is not a good day-by-day practice.

Some women claim that they can't face the light of day until they have their false lashes fixed in place. A few wake-up exercises performed in bed, we think, is a better start for any day. However, false lashes can be flattering, and for women of any age.

Lashes come in such categories as ''natural,'' ''shaggy,'' ''demi,'' ''half lashes,'' etc. Normally, upper and lower lashes come on a clear strip of plastic which is put on the eyelid and held in place by a special glue. Few women can wear lower lashes successfully. A number use the lower lashes on the upper lids, discarding the long, upper lashes. A better technique is to apply the long lashes to your upper lids, choose a length that looks as if you might have grown the lashes yourself, remove the lashes and then cut them to the desired length. Some women trim their lashes on their eyes. If you do that, take care. You don't want a horrible accident. If you have never worn artificial lashes and want to try out the effect, you might consider starting with half lashes.

Color? Your own natural color is usually best, but even if your hair is black, dark brown lashes are usually a better choice. Black lashes look fine on a black woman or on most Orientals, but for most Caucasians they are too dark. Their effect is aging.

MASCARA

Mascara is the only eye makeup used by some women. It comes in a variety of types—regular, waterproof, and ''eyelash extending.'' The color should match your own natural color as nearly as possible. If your eyelashes are exceedingly pale, then you might choose a light brown. For the majority of women, light brown to dark brown to black will be the choice. Apply two coats to the upper lashes, waiting a full five minutes between coats. Use mascara on the lower lashes sparingly—if at all. Properly chosen and carefully applied, mascara can really dramatize young eyes and contribute drama and a youthful look for the older woman.

Twenty

❧ANTI-WRINKLE WAYS TO BATHE❧

If we didn't wear clothes we would rarely be troubled by skin disease or odor, but our bodies, constantly exposed to the elements, particularly the sun, would wrinkle faster. At that, our bodies rarely emit an odor if our internal environment is healthy. Our diet usually affects how we smell, or *if* we smell. Orientals often are shocked by the smell of meat-eating Caucasians. Caucasians often are startled by the smell of certain Africans, unfortunately often attributing the odor to inadequate bathing rather than the true cause: difference in diet.

The odor from perspiration is often due to a combination of inadequate bathing, nerves, and activity. When perspiration is induced for any reason, effort should be made to bathe as soon thereafter as possible—for the sake of the skin, to rid it of the wastes eliminated through the perspiration, and to avoid offending by body odor.

Though it has become customary to bathe once a day, there are genuine benefits in bathing twice daily—if the water is not too hot and if the soap is *thoroughly* rinsed away. A "three bath" routine is suggested:

MORNING

"Dry scrub" with a loofah or a natural bristle bath brush or coarse terry towel to stimulate the circulation and help rid the skin of dry cells. Follow this with a "wake-up shower": warm water shifting to tepid or cold, or alternating warm and cold water. Choose a gentle, well-fatted soap, and rinse well. A cold splash, or alternating warm-cold showers, will impart a sense of well-being and give the skin a

163

lovely glow. A cold bath or shower may not sound attractive, but if you try it once, you'll find that it's enjoyable and is conducive to a lasting sense of well-being and aliveness. If your skin turns blue instead of pink, you have stayed in the cold water too long, or the temperature was simply too cold for you. Healthy pink is the goal.

For the person in less than good health, a cold sponge bath with cloth or sponge, is a good alternative and provides similar benefits.

Dry with a medium weight towel. Many of the most luxurious towels seem to rub *over* rather than absorbing moisture, and can be too heavy for many women to handle with ease. Choose big bath towels. A skimpy towel may dry, but certainly imparts no psychological values of feeling pampered and special.

NIGHT

If you wish, take an alternating hot-cold foot bath as a preliminary to your bath. Such a foot bath is a great aid to circulation.

For your bath, use pleasantly warm water to which you have added a tablespoon or two of cold-pressed vegetable or seed oil—corn or sesame or sunflower. The oil will give the skin a silky feeling. Or you may choose a different additive, or none.

WEEKLY

An epsom salt bath will stimulate the skin and relax the muscles. The water should be fairly hot. About 98° to 100° is usually right. Use one-half pound to three pounds of salts, depending upon the size of your tub and the amount of water you use. Soap up to 30 minutes, adding hot water as desired.

Finish with a tepid rinse or shower. After toweling dry, lavish the arms, legs, and body with a good creamy lotion or oil.

Bath Additives

The state and quality of your skin should be your guide as to whether you put anything into the bath water. Basically, there are three types of additives: bath oils, bath salts, and bubble baths.

OILS

Commercial oils contain oil, perfume, water, soap or detergent, and sometimes a small amount of alcohol or other preservative. These oils leave a film that softens the skin. An oil from a supermarket or health food store may be preferred by many—and will cost less. It may be better to avoid perfume and alcohol, especially if you are allergy-prone. If your skin is inclined to be dry, oil should be your choice. Try to avoid bath oils with mineral oil in them. A friend confessed to us that she uses corn oil, or Crisco when showering, or some other cooking shortening.

SALTS

Many use bath salts simply because these perfume the water or add a pleasant color tone, but the basic purpose is to soften hard water, to counteract the minerals to allow soap to cleanse more efficiently. When the water is very hard, the soap fails to lather effectively and leaves a sticky film on the skin and hair.

Bath salts consist of a salt, such as sodium carbonate, plus a perfume and some kind of coloring agent. While removing excess salt from the water, bath salts can be drying to the skin. If the water in your area is hard and you use bath salts, you should apply body lotion or oil to your skin after your bath.

BUBBLES

The primary purpose of putting a bubble bath product into the water is for glamour—to impart a sense of luxury, a feeling of being pampered. The benefit therefore is primarily psychological. Bubbles are made with a sulfur-derivative detergent, water, dye, and perfume. Generally they don't soften water or skin, and they can be irritating, not only to the skin but to the delicate tissues of the vagina. While all right for an agreeable, occasional treat, ''bubbles'' should not be a routine addition to your bath water.

Post-Bath Skin Aids

The purpose of the after-bath lotions and powders is to soothe and smooth the skin and sometimes to nourish or cool it.

BODY LOTIONS AND OILS

These are recommended for the normal or dry skin. Besides the good commercial lotions and oils available, you can make excellent ones yourself at little cost. Recipes are in the Appendix.

BATH POWDERS

Like lotions and oils, bath powders are designed to make your skin feel soft and silky, and, in the case of commercial powders, to perfume it. Powders are often the first choice when the skin is inclined to be oily. Powder is particularly agreeable in the summer, since it feels cooling on application. Scents range from delicate florals to exotic "orientals." Or you can buy Fuller's Earth or rice powder in most pharmacies. You can pulverize rice and sift it through a linen handkerchief; perfumed with your own special scent, it is truly individual.

ROUGH SPOTS

Rub the skin with a handful of wet cornmeal to "sand" the rough spots from elbows, thighs, and other parts of the skin. Rough skin that catches on hose and that always feels scuffy is truly unpleasant—for those who touch you as well as yourself. The elder flower was used in Victorian times to smooth skin, but today, careful washing with a grainy substance, and then application of a soothing oil such as sesame oil, or applying some other lotion will help. Often, rough skin tells you that some substance that you are using is irritating to you; you have an allergic reaction. The best defense is probably to avoid that substance—whether it is soap, wool, or perfume.

Handy Tools

A *bath thermometer* should almost be considered an essential so that you can use your bath for greatest effectiveness and with greatest ease. Choose temperatures from cool to a ''normal'' 92° to 96°, to a muscle-easing or therapeutic hot bath that may range from 98° to 108°.

A *bath tray* that hooks across the tub to hold such items as a small stand-up mirror is useful. The tub is a good place to tweeze your eyebrows or exercise or massage your face. The tray also can hold such items as a pumice stone to attack scaly elbows or heels, or a bowl of cornmeal.

Loofahs come in many sizes and shapes. A loofah is a plant fiber that expands upon immersion in water. A long loofah can be favored for ''dry scrubs'' and for use in the shower, whereas you might prefer a loofah mitt for use in the bath.

Natural sponges are a pleasant way to soap the body, particularly in the bath.

Washcloths seem more utilitarian than sponges and are a problem in that, in most homes, they are overused. A washcloth should be used only once for the bath or the face, and then should be laundered.

Loofahs and sponges should be rinsed in very hot water after use.

Plastic mitts and *brushes* often are promoted for stimulating and exfoliating the skin, but they should be avoided. They can scratch and pull the skin, and in addition to being injurious, they encourage wrinkles.

Anti-Wrinkle Bathing Techniques: Summary

Use warm water routinely, shifting to cool or cold for brief periods.

Always dry *upward* if you are toweling yourself at all.

Oil in the bath water will leave your skin feeling silky.

Pleasant music can be a decidedly enjoyable and beneficial accompaniment for prebed or preparty bathing.

Reading in the tub is not conducive to relaxation and should be avoided. Regular periods of relaxation, including time in the tub, should be a basic element of your anti-wrinkle program.

You may not desire to hold court while taking your bath as did certain famous beauties of history (and some even in current times), but you definitely should consider your bath time as special, designed to make you feel good mentally as well as physically, and to contribute toward your anti-wrinkle goals.

Twenty-one

🌿ANTI-WRINKLE BEAUTY FOODS IN YOUR DIET AND ON YOUR SKIN🌿

Skin care wasn't invented in the twentieth century. Beauties from the most ancient time, the most primitive societies, always have been concerned with keeping their skin lovely and preventing wrinkles. Their aids included olive oil and other oils from seeds, plants, and flowers; herbs from the garden; and many fruits and vegetables.

Until recently, it was claimed that no skin product would penetrate the skin. That is true when mineral oil is a key ingredient. Mineral oil is an inhibitor of penetration: it sits on the skin and leaches moisture from it. On the other hand, it has been reported that a component of polyunsaturated oil penetrates the skin within ten minutes.

Apricots, papayas, cherries, tomatoes, raspberries, grapes, carrots, bananas, lemons, strawberries, cucumbers, and avocados are delicious, beauty-giving foods in the diet, and beauty aids for the skin.

Some fruits and vegetables will cleanse the skin. Others nourish it. Fruits contribute their vitamins, minerals, pectins, and humectant, the element that supplies moisture to the skin and helps it stay moist.

169

The inside of the peeling of some fruits will help exfoliate the skin, to rid it of dead cells. The inside of the peel of the papaya will do this, and pineapple juice is an exfoliator too. The skin's ability to shed the outer surface diminishes as years accumulate. Destruction of the normal acid mantle of the skin also seems to slow down the process by which the skin sheds its outer layer. Fruit juice extracts have an acid reaction which is beneficial to maintenance of the normal pH of the skin; the normal pH is more acid than alkaline, approximately in the ratio of 6 to 5.2.

Beauties of ancient Rome used grapes on their skin to discourage wrinkles. When preparing fruits and vegetables for use on your skin, keep in mind that these products keep no longer than they do as food. After preparation, and between use, ''homemade'' beauty treatments should be refrigerated since they contain no preservatives. Make up only small amounts so that they can be used up right away. That's the best way to prepare food you eat, too. Leftovers always are less rich in nutrients.

Avocado

Avocados, used by the ancient Aztecs to moisturize the skin and give body to the hair, are perhaps the most versatile of all beauty foods.

They contain 73 percent moisture in a natural emulsification, eight vitamins and seven essential minerals. Unlike most fruits, they also contain a small amount (2 percent) of protein.* Skin and hair respond wonderfully to the abundant vitamins, minerals, and precious oil of the avocado. As a hair conditioner, the avocado brings new life to thirsty locks. They're particularly valuable for sun- or wind-damaged skin.

Use only fully ripe avocados. Several grooming recipes call for mashed, pureed, or macerated avocado pulp. To prepare, peel the skin

---

*Other fruits containing protein include apricots (1.6 grams per cup fresh, raw; 6.5 grams per cup dried), oranges (1.8 grams per medium orange), red raspberries (1.5 grams per cup), black raspberries (2 grams per cup), uncooked prunes (2.3 grams per ten dried prunes).

and remove pit. Use fork, blender, potato ricer, food mill, or sieve to mash or puree. Avocados are perishable. Some formulas are designed for one-time use only, others may be refrigerated for 48 hours.

Every part of the fruit can be used as a beauty aid. The avocado is the base for many preparations. The inside of the peel is rich in oil. Rub it vigorously on hands and feet to lubricate rough skin. The cleaned seed is an excellent facial exerciser for the throat. It will fit right into your hand, and its shape and texture are perfect for massaging any of the avocado recipes into the skin. The pit also can be placed in avocado mixtures to help prevent darkening of the pulp, which occurs naturally from exposure to air. In food recipes, darkening is usually prevented by the addition of lemon or lime juice, but these citrus juices may be too harsh for some dry or sensitive skins.

Avocado skin color will vary with the seasons, from brilliant leaf green, through hunter's green, to deep violet and brown-black. The nourishment is identical.

AVOCADO FACIAL CLEANSER

Yolk of 1 egg
½ cup milk (fresh milk or reconstituted dry milk)
½ ripe avocado, peeled and mashed

- Put all in a blender, if you have one, or beat together until you have a thin cream or a lotionlike consistency. Apply to the skin with balls of cotton or gauze squares. Work as you would any cream; rinse with tepid water, and then cool water. Dry face carefully.

This cleanser can be used after ordinary soap and water cleansing, if your skin is normal, or, if your skin is sensitive to all soaps, the avocado cleanser is effective in itself against pollution and grime.

Since the formula is perishable, a recipe should be made up every other day and stored in the refrigerator between uses.

171

AVOCADO/CORNMEAL FACIAL SCRUB

½ ripe avocado, peeled and mashed
½ cup cornmeal

- Blend the two together well. Apply the avocado/cornmeal paste to your fresh-cleansed face. Scrub gently with a circular motion. This will slough off dead tissue and is a super-cleanser. Rinse the face well with tepid water to remove. Finishing touch: a splash of cold witch hazel. This scrub is excellent for rough skin.

AVOCADO NIGHT CREAM

1 teaspoon ripe avocado
1 teaspoon favorite night cream

- Mash the avocado and blend with night cream. Massage the cream into the skin gently, using upward, outward movements. You can use your fingers, palms of your hands, or the avocado seed. Remove after 20 minutes or allow to remain on skin all night.

AVOCADO ANTI-WRINKLE CREAM

½ avocado, pureed
1 tablespoon fresh wheat germ

- Blend the two together. Rub the cream into the neck and jawline areas with firm strokes. The vitamin E in the avocado will penetrate the skin's surface and stimulate the tissue and muscles underneath. You can use this cream with our ''smoothings'' technique with great benefit. Used nightly, the cream, with smoothings, produces most spectacular results.

AVOCADO TREATMENT FOR PUFFY EYES

½ avocado, peeled and sliced into quarter-inch crescents

- Lie down on bed or slant board and secure a few slices of avocado under each eye. (You can use transparent tape.) Rest for about 20 minutes. Corrective magic.

AVOCADO MASQUE MARVELS

For large pores and sallowness

½ avocado, mashed
1 tablespoon honey
¼ cup milk, at room temperature

- Mix together (with fork or blender) until thoroughly blended. Clean the face, neck, chest, and shoulders thoroughly, including back of neck using your favorite method. Apply the mixture and lie down and rest for 20 minutes. Remove with tepid water only or use water with a sponge or clean washcloth. Follow with a brisk patting of cool water.

For dry skin:

Yolk of 1 egg
½ avocado

- Beat the yolk until light and frothy. Mash the avocado. Mix the two together with fork or in blender. Spread the mixture on a thoroughly clean face and throat and relax on bed or slant board for 20 minutes. Remove with tepid water. Rinse with cold water. Use weekly.

For oily skin:

White of 1 egg
1 teaspoon lemon juice
½ avocado

- Put all ingredients into a blender. On a very clean face, apply the masque and relax for 20 minutes. Remove with tepid water. Follow with a splash of ice cold astringent or skin tonic.
- If your skin is *very* oily, you can precede the masque by using the avocado-cornmeal scrub on your face.

173

SPECIAL OCCASION MASQUE

2 tablespoons instant nonfat dry milk

2 tablespoons water

½ peeled, ripe avocado, mashed smooth

- Mix the milk and water into a smooth, thick paste in a small bowl. Work in the avocado with a fork. Apply a portion of this to a clean face and throat. When you begin to feel your skin stiffening, add another layer. When that dries, in about 10 minutes, remove the masque with tepid water and a sponge or clean washcloth. Rinse well with clear water. Follow with a commercial skin freshener or fruit wash.

ANTI-WRINKLE MASQUE

Cake of yeast

1 to 1 ½ tablespoons whole milk or cream

¼ avocado, pureed

- Mash the cake of yeast until it dissolves in the milk. Add the avocado. Blend well. Apply mixture to a clean face and neck, avoiding the eye area since the masque exerts considerable pull as it dries.
- The yeast will draw impurities from the skin, the vitamin-rich avocado will lubricate it, and the milk or cream will bring out a glow.
- Remove the masque with warm water and a sponge or clean washcloth. Follow with cold water, skin tonic, or astringent.

HALF-HOUR MASQUE

¼ avocado, pureed

1 teaspoon olive, almond, or sesame oil

White of 1 egg, beaten to a froth

1 teaspoon honey

- Blend oil and avocado and massage into the skin of face and neck, upward and outward for 5 minutes. When the skin has absorbed as much as it can, remove the excess lightly with a soft tissue.

- Stir honey into egg white and apply to skin over the remaining avocado and oil. Relax on bed or slant board for 20 minutes while the egg white and honey masque dries on the skin, tightening the pores in the process.
- Use warm water to remove the masque. Follow with cold water and a fruit rinse.

ANTI-BROWN SPOTS MASQUE

This masque helps brighten the skin after a summer tan begins to fade. It can also help lighten freckles and brown spots—but patience is required.

½ avocado, mashed
Rind of ½ lemon, grated fine
1 teaspoon lemon juice

- Mix the three together in a bowl and massage into the skin for a few minutes. Leave on for about 15 minutes. Remove the excess. The residue may be left on overnight.
- If the skin is very dry, remove the cream after 5 minutes, rinse with warm, followed by cool, water.

AVOCADO SCALP TREATMENT

Yolk of 1 egg
½ avocado, thoroughly mashed
1 teaspoon lemon juice
½ cup of olive, sesame, almond, safflower, or soybean oil

- In a warm bowl, beat the egg yolk slightly with a wire whisk. Add a small amount of oil, beat. Add the avocado slowly and then add the remainder of the oil, a teaspoon at a time, beating after each addition. Add the lemon juice.
- Beat to blend well.
- This should make about one cup, which will keep a few days if refrigerated. Apply the concoction to the hair taking a thin strand of hair at a time, saturate it, especially the ends, with the mixture. Then apply the remaining treatment to the scalp,

massaging in well. Allow it to remain on the hair for at least half an hour or, better, overnight. (Wrap your head in a towel to protect bed linen.)

- Follow with a shampoo, first rinsing hair and head with warm water and then gradually adding shampoo. Work your hair and scalp with your hands until you get a good lather. Two applications of shampoo may be required to remove the avocado-oil conditioner.

- For damaged or dyed hair, use twice weekly to start. Even the driest and most abused hair will take on new luster and manageability with this beauty treatment. After results begin to show, a semi-monthly treatment will be adequate.

Bananas

Bananas are believed to be the most ancient of fruits yet they are relatively new to North America. Alexander the Great found bananas growing when he invaded India. They were the favorite food of holy men, a fact which earned them the name, ''the fruit of the wise men.''

Anyone seeking health and beauty is wise to include bananas in the diet. They are comparatively low in calories—only 85 for a six-inch fruit—and they contain 22.2 grams of complex carbohydrate (the kind that's good for you), calcium, phosphorus, iron, sodium, potassium, and vitamins A, B_1, B_2, B_6, C, and niacin.

The banana is a fiber-rich food and so is important for the elimination of constipation. It is important in diabetics' diets, and is often recommended specifically for sufferers from colitis, peptic ulcer, and gastric disorders. A number of investigators have attributed the fruit's effectiveness to its pectin, which swells, causing soft, bland stools that clear the intestinal tract. Pectin also aids in eliminating infectious bacteria and promoting growth of beneficial bacteria.

The banana can help promote skin beauty from the outside, too, and its low cost makes it feasible to use even all over the body as a prebath beauty treatment, particularly when blended with ripe avocado.

AVOCADO/BANANA PREBATH SKIN CREAM

1 ripe banana, peeled
1 ripe avocado, peeled and pitted

- Put both fruits through a potato ricer. Press well so that the two blend thoroughly. Rub the mixture all over the body or on only those areas where the skin needs nourishment to eliminate dryness. For best results, leave on one hour before rinsing, showering, or bathing off.
- If only a small amount is used, the remainder may be stored in the refrigerator, with the pit of the avocado embedded in the mixture to prevent discoloration. It's a good idea to cover the bowl with plastic wrap.

Cucumber

''Cool as a cucumber'' is more than just a phrase. Cucumbers seem actually cooling to the system when eaten during hot summer days. In India it is common practice to pass a bowl of sliced cucumbers following a hot, spicy meal.

Cucumbers are used around the world in the diet and on the skin, as a refiner, purifier, and refresher.

Many women simply rub their faces with slices of cucumber, finding it helpful in such varied situations as oily skin, troubled skin, or end-of-day fatigue.

CUCUMBER MASQUE #1

1 cucumber, cut up
3 ounces skim or low-fat milk

- Put the cucumber and milk into the blender and liquify.
- Apply the mixture to your face, throat, neck, arms, chest.
- Allow to remain 10 to 15 minutes, wash off, and then rinse. Your skin and the rest of you will feel refreshed.

CUCUMBER MASQUE #2

½ cup chopped cucumber
2 teaspoons powdered milk
White of 1 egg

- Blend ingredients into a paste and apply to neck and face in upward, outward motions. Allow masque to dry for 30 minutes. Rinse off with warm water. Finish with cool water. Pat face dry.

CUCUMBER/AVOCADO MASQUE

½ cucumber, peeled and finely chopped
½ avocado, peeled and mashed

- Press out the juice from the cucumber through a fine sieve or piece of cheesecloth, and reserve the juice for Cucumber Lotion (below). Mix the cucumber pulp with the avocado. Apply to a thoroughly clean neck and face and leave on for 15 minutes. Remove with tepid water. Rinse with cool. Finish by briskly patting face with Cucumber Lotion.

CUCUMBER LOTION

Simply pat the face with cucumber juice. If any is left over, store it in the refrigerator until the next time you wish to use it.

Papaya

Papaya is a wonderful fruit, superb to taste, an aid to digestion, soothing to the upset stomach, cleansing to the intestines, and beautifying for the skin. Papaya is a better source of vitamin C than orange juice, is rich in vitamin A, a fair source of vitamin B, and a

178

good source of vitamin G. It contains an enzyme that aids digestion and assimilation of protein, and some of the fats and starches. Natives of tropical countries, where papaya grows, wrap tough meat in papaya leaves to soften it—a practice that led to manufacture of various meat tenderizers with a papaya base.

Women in the tropics rub their skin with papaya fruit to remove freckles, blemishes, and brown spots, and to soften the skin. After eating the fruit, rub the inside of the papaya skin on your clean face. It softens and smoothes.

Pineapple

Fresh pineapple is a delightful fruit when eaten in itself, it can be cooked with ham and poultry, and it is versatile in salads and in desserts. The bromelain enzyme in fresh pineapple reputedly aids the action of antibiotics, and it's a skin aid too. It actually dissolves the top layer of dead cells. To put the pineapple's exfoliating action to work, create a . . .

FRESH PINEAPPLE WASH

This works easiest if you have a juicer. Put chunks of pineapple through the juicer until you have ¼ cup. Saturate double thicknesses of gauze or cheesecloth with the pineapple juice, and relax on the bed or a slant board for 15 minutes with the pineapple-soaked gauze covering your face and throat. (If you feel that the full-strength fruit juice is too strong, you can dilute it a little with spring, distilled, or boiled water.)

Rinse your face with warm water. Rub face gently with sponge or a soft natural bristle brush to rid the skin of dead cells. Be gentle to avoid irritation. Rinse again in warm and then cool water. Blot the skin dry. Smooth on a favorite cream.

AVOCADO/PINEAPPLE MASQUE

½ avocado, peeled

1 tablespoon *fresh* pineapple juice (see recipe above)

- While you mash the avocado, slowly add the pineapple juice.
  (If fresh pineapple juice is not obtainable, use canned,
  unsweetened juice.) Apply the ''cream'' to a thoroughly
  clean face and throat and massage it in well but gently. Relax
  for 10 minutes. Remove with cotton pads soaked in fresh
  pineapple juice. Follow with fresh cool water. Pat dry.
  The bromelain enzyme in the pineapple juice will exfoliate
  dead skin cells while the avocado will oil and nourish the
  skin.

Strawberries

In the diet, strawberries contribute vitamins A and C and a number of
minerals, including potassium, calcium, and phosphorus. Also, since
their pH is the same as that of our skin, they can be a particular beauty
aid when used on the skin.

STRAWBERRY SKIN SOFTENER

1 cup ripe strawberries

1 cup spring or distilled water

- An old beauty treatment: mash the sun-ripened strawberries
  in the water. Before retiring, apply to the face, throat, arms,
  shoulders, bosom, and hands. The strawberries soften the
  skin and aid the exfoliating process. Wash away the dried
  mixture in the morning. ''Tired skin'' seems to go with it.

STRAWBERRY MASQUE

Wash and hull a handful of fresh, ripe strawberries, and with a
wooden spoon, mash them into a glass custard cup. Pat the straw-
berry juice over neck and face. Allow to dry. Rinse away with tepid
water.

If your skin is sensitive, blend in an equal amount of water before applying to the skin.

STRAWBERRY AND CREAM MASQUE

Mash several fresh, washed strawberries in a glass custard cup. Mix in an equal amount of fresh, rich cream. When the two are well blended, smooth onto the face, using tapping movements, upward on the neck, upward and outward on the face.

• Relax on a bed or slant board for 30 minutes. Rinse the mixture away with tepid water. Finish with cold.

POST-SUMMER MASQUE WITH STRAWBERRIES

½ cup ripe strawberries, washed and hulled
½ avocado, peeled and mashed

• Press strawberries through a sieve into a custard cup. Blend with avocado. On a clean face and throat, massage the strawberry-avocado masque into the skin for 3 minutes.
• Relax for 10 minutes. Remove with a damp, clean washcloth.
• Rinse with clear, cool water.
• This masque helps restore the skin after exposure to too much wind or sun.

STRAWBERRY ROSE LOTION

1 cup fresh, ripe, washed strawberries
4 ounces rose water (obtainable at your pharmacy)

• Using a sieve, press the juice out of the strawberries into a small bowl. Add the rose water. Chill before use, or add an ice cube to the mixture before you pat it on your face. Leave it on for 10 minutes. Rinse with clear water. Or the lotion may be left on all night to condition your skin while you sleep.
The lotion will keep for about two days in the refrigerator.

181

Other lotions you can use:

PEACHES AND CREAM

½ fresh, ripe peach, mashed
Fresh whole milk, or, better, rich cream

- Blend a few drops of milk or cream into fresh peach pulp and smooth on face to awaken skin to a happy glow.

PEAR RUB

Ripe pears are beneficial when applied to oily or blemished skin. After cleansing the face thoroughly, rub with a cut side of the fruit. Keep the substance on the face 15 minutes, or, for a particularly blemished condition, overnight. The pear has a disinfecting action.

WATERMELON LOTION

When watermelons are in season, make a watermelon lotion to wake up your skin. Cut a slice of a chilled, ripe watermelon, cut off the rind, and force the fruit through a sieve. Strain the juice. Pat on the face. Allow it to dry for about 5 minutes, then rinse off with clear, cold water.

Twenty-two

ANTI-WRINKLE WAYS TO SLEEP

You can create or combat wrinkles by the way you sleep. Most of us were taught to sleep on our right sides. If we slept on our left, we were told, it put an extra burden on the heart. If we slept on our back, we had nightmares.

Tell that to an elderly Japanese who traditionally slept on his back on a wooden neck board, and he will probably look at you in puzzlement. In recent years, sleep science has come into being and taught us we shift our positions often during a night's sleep. However, if you are among the majority who learned to sleep on your right, if you have wrinkles, you are likely to find your right cheek more wrinkled than your left.

As the best wrinkle preventive and wrinkle cure, borrow from the ancient Japanese. Sleep on your back. Instead of following the traditional Japanese way of sleeping on a mat and quilt on the floor, use the firmest possible mattress. If you were trained from childhood to believe back-sleeping will cause nightmares, when you go to bed you should fix in your mind that you are going to have happy, healthy, rest-producing dreams.

And throw away your thick pillows. Thick pillows are conducive to neck wrinkles, facial wrinkles, and hollows under the eyes. Use a baby pillow of down, unless you are allergic to feathers, or thin foam unless you are allergic to foam.

Don't sleep in an embryonic position. Sleep stretched out.

If you must sleep on your side, don't put your hand under your cheek. That causes wrinkles.

Don't sleep with your head fallen forward toward your chest. That causes wrinkles.

Don't sleep with your shoulders curled forward. That causes your bosom to sag and inhibits intake of oxygen. Sleep with your shoulders back.

If the weather is very cold and your feet are cold, you can heat your bed with a heating pad or electric blanket, but it's not best for you to sleep all night long with such aids. Warm your feet in a hot foot bath, or alternating hot and cold, to stimulate the circulation so that you will feel warm in the chilliest weather.

The amount of exercise you get during the day, the character of your daily nutrition, and your general mental state are basic factors in the quality of your rest. You cannot rest well if you have a distillery within you pumping gas and toxic materials into your bloodstream all night. As you exercise more, and thereby aid assimilation and elimination, you will require fewer hours in bed because the hours you do spend will be truly beneficial.

If insomnia strikes, don't bother counting sheep. Do any relaxing exercise at the *slowest* possible speed, counting the movement slowly. The monotony of it all will induce sleep. Garlic— swallowed raw or cooked and eaten in foods, or taken in capsule form —has been scientifically proven to reduce and eventually end insomnia for many persons.

The goal of truly beneficial sleep requires that you eliminate the destructive habit of making worry your bed companion. It is trite but true that most of what we worry about never happens. Recognize what a thief worry is of your happiness and rest—and what an enemy it is of your goal of being forever wrinkle free.

Twenty-three

☙TEN-DAY ANTI-WRINKLE PROGRAM☙

How much time should you give to yourself for a complete beauty program? Why, time enough for a new pattern of health to last you a lifetime.

Right now you spend one-third of your life in bed, too often sleeplessly. An hour a day devoted to exercise and to improving your circulation, muscles, and appearance will help you sleep like a baby, increase your efficiency, and produce benefits without number in your life. We urge you, therefore, to make a ten-day trial, at the very least, to devote one hour a day to becoming younger, healthier, happier, and more beautiful. We anticipate, of course, that you will be so delighted with the benefits of these ten hours that thereafter you will feel you deserve *and need* one hour a day to help yourself make the most of yourself. Here is your daily routine for ten days:

On awakening: Perform as many of the ''Exercises to Do in Bed'' as possible (Chapter 17) and as many of the other lying-down exercises—to be done in bed or on the floor or slant board—as you desire.

On arising: Give your eyes a clear water or chlorophyll eye bath (see Appendix for recipe).

Drink a glass of hot water to raise the blood temperature to aid digestion of breakfast. *Optional:* Add two ounces of prune juice or the juice of half a lemon. *Optional:* Swallow a clove of raw garlic (cut it into two or three pieces if it's large). Don't chew it! Swallow it with

185

a little water; *in the beginning* follow by chewing a sprig of parsley or watercress to kill the odor. *Optional:* Devote 10 to 20 minutes to meditation or prayer. A wise man said: ''When we pray to God, we talk to Him. When we meditate, we listen.''

Before breakfast: Spend 10 to 30 minutes on facial cleansing, facial exercise, nourishment (creaming), smoothings, and makeup.

Breakfast.

Mid-morning: Have a vitamin/mineral-rich snack.

Lunch.

After lunch: If possible, wash your face with soap and water, rinse well (25 to 50 times), pat dry, spray with ''lemon water,'' and apply moisturizer. Allow the skin to absorb the moisturizer at least five minutes if you follow with makeup.

Late afternoon: Have a snack—fruit, nuts, or seeds.

Before dinner: Devote 30 minutes to predinner beauty routines, relax by lying flat on your back on a firm bed or even the floor. *Note:* If you give yourself a beauty masque during this period, you can keep your face agreeably relaxed while performing a number of simple exercises, such as exercising (see Part 5). Don't do facial exercises while you have on any kind of facial masque. Keep your face still and serene.

Dinner.

Evening: A carrot stick, a small apple, or a half of a pear makes a nice, easy-to-digest snack if you are hungry.

Before bedtime: Wash your face with soap and water. Rinse 25 to 30 times. Perform facial exercises and smoothings. Give yourself a dry body rub to rid the skin of dead cells (see Chapter 20). Take a bath, adding one or two tablespoons of pure vegetable or seed oil to the bath water. You can perform many eye and foot and leg exercises while soaking in tub.

Sleep well! Happy dreams!

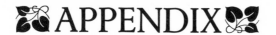 APPENDIX

Dietary Aids

APPLE/HERB DRINK

1 teaspoon dandelion root
1 teaspoon angelica
1 teaspoon wormwood
1 teaspoon gentian
2 cups water (distilled or spring)
2 quarts freshly squeezed apple juice
4 ounces freshly squeezed lemon juice

- Simmer dandelion, angelica, wormwood, and gentian in water for 10 minutes. Strain. Add apple and lemon juices.
- Drink concoction in small portions throughout the day for two days while confining diet during that period to stewed fruit and/or apple juice. *Do not fast without* your *doctor's permission.*
- Repeat, if needed, once monthly.
- In time, according to a famous medical authority, an added bonus with this drink is that brown spots will disappear from hands.
- Don't ignore the role of chewing in providing anti-wrinkle exercise for the throat, jaw, mouth, and cheek muscles. Crunchy raw vegetables—including raw carrots, raw rutabaga, and leafy greens—provide exercise as well as valuable nutrients. So does:

CORN PONE BREAKFAST EXERCISER

2 cups cornmeal
¾ teaspoon salt
3 tablespoons shortening
1 ⅓ cups boiling water

- Combine cornmeal and salt in mixing bowl. Stir in shortening and water. Mix thoroughly. Cover pan with a cloth. Let stand 15 to 30 minutes. Moisten hands with oil and form dough into 12 to 15 flat cakes. Bake on a greased cookie sheet 35 to 40 minutes in oven preheated to 350°.

• These cakes are nutritious for breakfast and excellent exercise for the throat and jaw muscles. Eating corn pone regularly should eliminate the most stubborn double chin.

• While you won't get the exercise benefit, you still gain the nutritional when you substitute corn pone crumbs in recipes calling for bread crumb topping. Put half a dozen of the corn cakes between two sheets of wax paper and use a rolling pin to crush them into crumbs. After spreading the crumbs over the vegetable, fish, or meat casserole, dot butter or margarine over the top.

ANTI-WRINKLE COCKTAIL

1 tablespoon safflower or sesame oil
2 tablespoons low-fat milk
3 tablespoons low-calorie coffee soda or 7-Up
1 vitamin E capsule

• Have all ingredients well chilled. Put into blender and run machine until the vitamin E capsule dissolves.

• One of these cocktails daily, preferably taken 30 minutes before a meal, will provide you with the polyunsaturated oil you need to help keep your cholesterol down and contribute to the healthy glow of your skin and gleam of your hair. The vitamin E will aid your skin and help you toward your youth-maintenance goals, and, as an anti-oxidant, it protects the oil.

• Polyunsaturated fatty acids are important for healthy skin and good metabolism and, some doctors believe, to healthy hearts. However, they are unstable compounds. The polyunsaturated fatty acid molecules can break down into particles that, when combined with oxygen molecules, will form toxic peroxides that can damage and destroy cells and encourage signs of aging.

• Putting the vitamin E capsule into the Anti-Wrinkle Cocktail is insurance against peroxidation damage. Whether the capsule you take represents 100, 200, or 400 International Units depends upon what your doctor recommends.

Beauty Aids

ANTI-FRECKLE LOTION

Handful of fresh elder flowers
Distilled or spring water to cover (or water that has been boiled one
hour and cooled)

- Allow to stand overnight. Strain. Bathe freckles (and brown
  spots) twice daily.

EYE WASHES

Wash eyes with distilled water.

ANTI-BLACKHEAD PASTE

Refined Fuller's Earth
Witch Hazel

- Make a paste of the two ingredients and smooth it over
  areas where blackheads occur. Leave it on your face until it
  flakes. Rinse off with tepid water. Pat dry. Follow, if
  desired, with an application of your favorite cream, lotion,
  or astringent.

Skin Creams and Lotions

THREE-OIL LOTION

1 ounce oil of sweet almonds
3 ounces sesame oil
½ teaspoon lanolin

- Blend together in a small steel pot. Dissolve over low heat.
  Cool. Use twice daily, in the morning apply under makeup,
  and before retiring around eyes and on neck. Store, between
  use, in a stoppered jar in the refrigerator.

LIQUID PROTEIN LOTION

3 ounces polyunsaturated vegetable oil

1 ounce predigested liquid collagen protein (health or drug store)

- Blend ingredients together. Before retiring, massage into skin with gentle, upward, outward motions. Leave on all night.
- Store, between use, in stoppered jar or bottle in the refrigerator. Stir before each use. This mixture has been known to help plump up tissues of the mouth and face.

MASSAGE AND OVERNIGHT CREAM

4 ounces distilled or spring water (or boiled, cooled tap water)

4 ounces comfrey leaves (dry or fresh) *or*

3 ounces comfrey root

4 ounces sesame oil

1 ounce predigested liquid collagen protein (health or drug store)

1 tablespoon liquid lecithin

1 tablespoon uncooked honey

- Bring water and comfrey to boil. Reduce heat. Simmer 5 minutes. Remove from heat. Cool. Strain. Blend with fork (not in blender) liquid protein and lecithin. Add 2 tablespoons strained comfrey tea. Blend with fork. Heat honey in a small jar in a small pan of water. Add heated honey to mixture.
- Stir well. Massage this cream onto a clean face three times daily. When using before bedtime, allow the skin to absorb the cream, then smooth on a second coating and let it remain, without massaging, overnight.

FOR WINTER-REDDENED HANDS, ROUGH ELBOWS

Blend powdered milk with tepid water to make lotion. Wash hands and elbows with the mixture. This treatment will improve the color and smoothness.

Masques

HERBAL MASQUES

4 ounces herb tea of your choice, cool.
Handful of bay leaves or eucalyptus leaves

- Put ingredients into blender. Mixture should be thick enough to adhere to the skin. If not, add additional leaves. Store in a cool, dark place 3 to 4 days. To use, lie on bed or slant board and pat mixture all over clean face and throat. Relax 10 to 20 minutes. Rinse off with tepid water.

KEFIR YEAST MASQUE

1 tablespoon kefir yeast
Distilled, spring, or boiled water to make paste

- Spread paste on face, avoiding eye area. Lie on bed or slant board for 10 to 20 minutes while mask dries on skin. Rinse with clear, tepid water. Your skin will feel super clean.

MILK MASQUE

1 egg white
1 heaping teaspoon powdered milk

- Stir powdered milk into unbeaten egg white. Mix to pudding consistency. Smooth mask on clean face, neck, and throat, from collarbone to hairline, avoiding the eye area. Lie down, relax, and think happy thoughts for 10 minutes so that mask will dry on face with upturned lips.
- To remove, hold clean, cool, wet washcloth over your face until all ''pull'' on the muscles stops. Now rinse off the mask with tepid water. Rinse thoroughly, at least 25 rinses, to remove all traces of mask. If every bit is not removed, the skin will have a ''glazed'' look. This mask helps lighten as well as tone and firm the skin. It can be used daily until the skin is in excellent condition, after which it could be used weekly.

MILK OF MAGNESIA MASQUE

• Spread Milk of Magnesia liberally over clean throat and face, from collarbone to hairline, avoiding the eye area. Lie on bed or slant board 15 minutes while the Milk of Magnesia draws impurities from the skin. To remove, spread another layer of Milk of Magnesia over the first. Remove with warm wet washcloth. Rinse face and neck well with tepid water.

• Heat a small amount of pure olive oil in a tiny steel saucepan to slightly above body temperature. Dip clean balls of absorbent cotton into heated oil and apply to throat and face with upward, outward motions. Allow skin to absorb the oil for 5 minutes. Blot off any residue.

MUMMY MASQUE

• We learned about this masque from a beauty expert and manufacturer of some excellent skin creams. You can put the masque on yourself, but it is much easier if someone does it for you. You should leave it on for a minimum of three hours. Some women, dedicated to preventing wrinkles or reversing them as quickly as possible, will leave the masque on for as long as 72 hours!

• Three hours work seeming miracles. Put on soft music and rest quietly, thinking happy thoughts, or sleep. Don't talk or eat. If you want to drink water or juice, use a straw, but it's better to take nothing so that there is no interference with the muscles.

BASIC MASQUE

3 tablespoons slippery elm powder (crush slippery elm with your hands or in small electric nut or coffee grinder)
3 tablespoons distilled, spring, or boiled water
1 teaspoon papaya juice

• Put the three ingredients in the top of a steel or glass double boiler (don't use aluminum or enamel) and allow to boil about 5 minutes. Strain through cheesecloth or a clean section of old nylon hose. Refrigerate. The mixture will almost gel.

• To this mixture, you can add any natural tightener to which you are not allergic: egg white (1 or 2), about ¼ cup of each of the following: refined Fuller's Earth, Brewer's Yeast, Kefir Yeast, or alum.
Next, you need:

Surgical gauze cut into triangles, measuring 1-inch, 1-inch, and ½-inch.
Additional uncut gauze, since you may wish to add some irregularly shaped pieces
Cold cream
½-inch flat, soft-hair paintbrush (from art supply or Japanese ''variety'' store)
Hot water or hot plate so that gelatinous masque can be kept warm (not hotter than 140°F.)
Container for gauze

• The masque can be applied in one, two, or three layers. Three layers is best. The masque is to be applied to the throat and face, but the eyes, mouth, and nostrils remain uncovered —for vision, breath and, if necessary, food, drink, and mumbled speech.
• If you are giving yourself a mummy masque, sit in front of a mirror. If you are being given the masque treatment, lie down on a bed or suitable table or untilted slant board. The directions that follow are given for someone else to apply the masque to you.
• Apply a liberal coating of cold cream to the eyebrows and along the hairline. With paintbrush, pick up half a brushful of masking solution and paint onto the skin above the upper eyelids to the edge of the natural fold and up to the underedge of the eyebrow. The coat should be fairly heavy.
• Pick up piece of gauze with the tip of the brush and lay it onto the skin above the upper eyelids, with ½-inch side toward the eye and in line with the natural fold of the upper lid. (Subject should not close eyes.)

- Place a second piece of gauze alongside the first, with a slight overlap. Place a third and, if necessary, a fourth piece of gauze until the skin above the upper eyelid is gauzed from nose to temple. Usually the gauze will adhere readily to the moist, gelatinous material. If not, hold the gauze with the blunt tip of an orangewood stick until it adheres. Paint these pieces of gauze with a coating of the gelatinous solution, pasting them down firmly.

- Repeat the process with the other over-eyelid area lid. Now apply the solution and gauze to the under-eye area— from nose to temple. (Leave one-eighth inch of clear skin between solution and gauze and rim of lower lid.) Paint the gauze with solution to make sure overlaps are held securely. (The gauze pieces should not be brought too close to the inner and outer corners of the eyes. This would hinder comfortable movement of eyelids.)

- Next apply solution over bridge of nose, between eyebrows. Progression from that point will depend upon the individual ''operator.'' However, a logical plan is to work up from the bridge of the nose to the hairline; then down one side of the forehead to the temple, and continue, a section at a time, until the entire face and under-chin are masked with one layer of gauze.

- Only a few pieces of gauze should be applied at a time, and then smoothed and pasted down with a top coat of the masking solution. Fit and trim the gauze neatly and comfortably around the nostrils. The mid-nose need not be gauzed.

- Around the mouth, align the bias edge of the gauze right up to the rim of the pink of the lips, but allow a little extra space at the corners of the mouth to permit fairly free movement for liquid feeding, drinking, and mumbled speech. The bias edge of the gauze should be arranged to face along the outer edge of the masque, and a little of the masking solution should extend beyond the masque. After completing the first layer, inspect it. If there are any loose edges, smooth and paint with masking solution.

194

- By the time the under-chin and the desired neck area are gauzed, the eyes and forehead are usually dry enough so that the second coat of solution-gauze-solution can be applied. The second and third layers are applied in the same manner as the first. However, the gauzes should be laid so as to overlap and interlock well with the lower layer.
- When any hot solution is used, the water content will gradually evaporate so that the solution becomes too thick. From time to time, as necessary, a tiny amount of water should be added with an eyedropper and stirred to keep an even consistency throughout the application of the masque. (The problem is avoided with a cold solution, but cold solutions do not offer the same degree of compressing/firming power.)
- The subject's features should be kept perfectly still and placid so as not to disturb the masque. Although a properly constructed masque is reasonably comfortable, it can become a little annoying as it dries and the compression/drawing power increases. The subject may read or even do mild exercises, but rest, to soothing music, or sleep, is most beneficial.
- Masking of the neck, arms, hands, shoulders, and other body areas requires the same type of procedure. However, it is most important that the subject remain still and not flex the body part being treated. For instance, with arms, it is usually best to mask only one arm at a time.

Resource List

Anti-Aging Creams or Products

Cellvita RNA Rejuvenating Cream

U.S. and Canadian health food stores or specialty shops
or
NYAL Products Ltd.
2051 Ambassador Drive
Windsor, Ontario, Canada N9C 3R5

Lift n' Toning Powder
with Aloe Vera n' Ginseng Activator

Aloe Vera Natural Skin Care Centers
or
Living International
3730 Cavalier Drive
Garland, Texas 75042

Exfoliating Cream

Bio Peeling Cream

Health food stores
or
M. J. Saffon Skin Care
301 East 79th Street
New York, New York 10021

Eye Cream for Contact Lens Wearers (and others)

Optica

Opticians, drug stores, health food stores
or
NYAL Products Ltd.
2051 Ambassador Drive
Windsor, Ontario, Canada, N9C 3R5

Eye Herbs

Hippocrates Health Institute
25 Exeter Street
Boston, Massachusetts 02116

☙BIBLIOGRAPHY❧

Adams, Catherine F., *Nutritive Value of American Foods in Common Units.* Washington, D.C.: Agricultural Research Service, United States Department of Agriculture.

Adams, Ruth, and Frank Murray, *Vitamin E, Wonder Worker of the '70's?* New York: Larchmont Press, 1971.

Ashley, Ruth, and Tess Kirby, *Dental Anatomy and Terminology,* for Self-Study and Classroom Use. New York: John Wiley & Sons, Inc., 1977.

Bates, W. H., M.D., *Better Eyesight Without Glasses.* New York: Pyramid Book, published by arrangement with Holt, Rinehart and Winston, 1970.

Bennett, Sanford, *Old Age, Its Cause and Prevention,* The Story of an Old Body and Face Made Young. Mokelumne Hill, Calif.: Health Research, 1912, reprinted 1963.

Bethel, May, *The Healing Power of Herbs.* North Hollywood, Calif.: Wilshire Book Company, 1968.

Brady, William, M.D., *An Eighty Year Old Doctor's Secrets of Positive Health.* Englewood Cliffs, N.J.: Prentice-Hall, Inc., 1961.

Bragg, Patricia, *The Bragg Hollywood Beauty Plan,* Health Science, P.O. Box 15000, Santa Ana, Calif.: 92705.

Brennan, Dr. R. O., with William C. Mulligan, *Nutrigenetics.* New York: M. Evans and Co., Inc., 1975.

Cantor, Alfred J., M.D., *Dr. Cantor's Longevity Diet:* How to Slow Down Aging and Prolong Youth and Vigor. West Nyack, N.Y.: Parker Publishing Company, Inc., 1967.

Carter, Mildred, *Helping Yourself with Foot Reflexology.* West Nyack, N.Y.: Parker Publishing Company, Inc., 1969.

Castleton, Virginia, *The Handbook of Natural Beauty.* Emmaus, Pa.: Rodale Press, Inc., 1975.

Chase, Dr. Alice, *Nutrition for Health.* West Nyack, N.Y.: Parker Publishing Company, Inc., 1954.

Chase, Deborah, *The Medically Based No-Nonsense Beauty Book.* New York: Alfred A. Knopf, 1975.

Cheraskin, E., M.D., D.M.D., W. M. Ringsdorf, Jr., D.M.D., and Arline Brecher, *Psychodietetics*, Food as the Key to Emotional Health. Toronto and New York: Bantam Books, 1974.

Clark, Linda, *Face Improvement Through Exercise and Nutrition*, A Pivot Original Health Book. New Canaan, Conn.: Keats Publishing Co., 1973.

Clark, Linda, and Yvonne Martine, *Health, Youth and Beauty Through Color Breathing*. Millbrae, Calif.: Celestial Arts, 1976.

Cobleigh, Ira U., *Live Young as Long as You Live*. New York: Award Books: London: Tandem Books, by arrangement with Association Press, 1969.

Craig, Marjory, *Facing Saving Exercises*, A 6-Day Plan Which Teaches You How to Naturally Lift the Sagging Muscles of the Face. New York: Random House, 1970.

Dahl, Arlene, *Always Ask a Man*, Arlene Dahl's Key to Femininity. Englewood Cliffs, N.J.: Prentice-Hall, Inc., 1965.

de Spain, June, *The Little Cyanide Cookbook*, Delicious Recipes Rich in Vitamin B_{17}. Westlake Village, Calif.: American Media, 1976.

Diagram Group, *Woman's Body*, An Owner's Manual. New York and London: Paddington Press, Ltd., 1977.

Douris, Larry, and Mark Timon, *Dictionary of Health and Nutrition*. New York: Pyramid Books, 1976.

Editors of *Consumer Reports*, *The Medicine Show*, Some Plain Truths About Popular Remedies for Common Ailments. Mount Vernon, N.Y.: Consumer Union, 1971.

Eichenlaub, John E., M.D., *Dr. Eichenlaub's Home Tonics and Refreshers for Daily Health and Vigor*. Englewood Cliffs, N.J.: Prentice-Hall, Inc., 1963.

Ewart, Charles D., *How to Enjoy Eating Without Committing Suicide*. New York: Simon & Schuster, Cornerstone Library Publications, 1971.

Feldenkrais, M., *Body and Mature Behavior*, A Study of Anxiety, Sex, Gravitation and Learning. Tel Aviv, Israel: ALEF Ltd., 1949.

Fillian, Barbie, and Lida Livingston, *Eat Yourself Thin, Secrets of Harbor Island Spas*, New York: Frederick Fell, Inc., 1977.

198

Frank, Dr. Benjamin, and Philip Miele, *Dr. Frank's No-Aging Diet*. New York: The Dial Press, 1976.

Franklyn, Robert Alan, M.D., with Helen Gould, *The Art of Staying Young*. New York: An Essandess Special Edition, Division of Simon & Schuster, Inc., by arrangement with Frederick Fell, Inc., 1968.

French, Chester D., *Papaya, the Melon of Health*. New York: Arco Publishing Company, Inc., 1972.

Halsell, Grace, *Los Viejos, Secrets of Long Life from the Sacred Valley*. Emmaus, Pa.: Rodale Press, Inc., 1976.

Hauser, Gaylord, *Mirror, Mirror on the Wall*. New York: Farrar, Straus, and Giroux, Inc., 1960.

Newbold, H. L., M.D., *Mega-Nutrients for Your Nerves*. New York: Peter H. Wyden, Publisher, 1975.

Ott, John N., *Health and Light*. New York: Pocket Books, 1976; Devin-Adair Edition, 1973.

Prudden, Bonnie, *How to Keep Slender and Fit After Thirty*. New York: Bernard Geis Associates, 1961, 1969.

Reichman, Stanley, M.D., *Instant Fitness, For Total Health an Immediate Commitment*. New York: Dell, 1976.

Reilly, Dr. Harold J., Ruth Hagy Brod, *The Edgar Cayce Handbook for Health Through Drugless Therapy*. New York: Macmillan Publishing Co., 1975.

"The Relationship Between Calories and Weight," and "The Calorie Expenditure of Various Activities," *Encyclopedia Britannica*.

R. A. Richardson, D.O., *Facial Wrinkles*. Mokelumne Hill, Calif.: Health Research, 1964.

Ronsard, Nicole, *Cellulite*, Those Lumps, Bumps and Bulges You Couldn't Lose Before. New York: Bantam Books, 1973.

Runge, Senta Maria, *Face Lifting by Exercise*, 6th ed., Los Angeles, Calif.: Allegro Publishing Company, 1974.

Sassoon, Beverly, and Vidal Sassoon, with Camille Duhe, *A Year of Beauty and Health*. New York: Simon & Schuster, 1975.

Schoen, Linda Allen, ed., *The AMA Book of Skin and Hair Care*.
Philadelphia: J. B. Lippincott Company, 1976.

Science of Life Books, *The Vitamins Explained Simply*. Science of Life
Books, 4-12 Tattersalls Lane, Melbourne, Victoria, Australia, 1975.

Shelmire, Bedford, Jr., M.D., *The Art of Being Beautiful at Any Age*.
New York: Warner Books, Inc., 1975.

Stonecypher, D. D., M.D., *Getting Older and Staying Young*. New York:
W. W. Norton & Co.: Toronto: George J. McLeod, Ltd., 1974.

Thomas, Clayton L., *Taber's Cyclopedic Medical Dictionary*. Philadelphia:
F. A. Davis Company, 1973.

Tilney, Frederick, *Young at 73—and Beyond*. New York: Information
Inc., 1968.

Traven, Beatrice, *The Complete Book of Natural Cosmetics*. New York:
Simon & Schuster, 1974.

Valeska, Lizallota, *Nature's Rejuvenating Principles*. New York: Carlton
Press, Inc., 1971.

Vogel, Dr. H. C. A., *The Liver:* The Regulator of Your Health. Geneva,
Switzerland: Bioforce-Verlag Teufen (AR), 1962.

von Furstenburg, Diane, *Diane von Furstenburg's Beauty Book.* New York:
Simon & Schuster, 1977.

Wade, Carlson, *Magic Minerals, Key to Better Health*. New York: Arco
Publishing Company, Inc., 1967.

Watanabe, Tadashi, D.Sc., *Garlic Therapy*. Tokyo: Japan Publications,
Inc., 1974.

Whitten, Ivah Bergh, *What Colour Means to You*. Ashingdon, Rochford,
England: The C. W. Daniel Company Ltd., 1963.

Wigmore, Dr. Ann, *Be Your Own Doctor*. Hippocrates Health Institute,
25 Exeter Street, Boston.

Williams, Roger J., *Nutrition Against Disease*. New York: Pitman
Publishing Corporation, 1971.

Zizmor, Jonathan, M.D., and John Foreman, *Superskin*, The Doctor's
Guide to a Beautiful Healthy Complexion. New York: Thomas Y.
Crowell Company, 1976.